the role of the brain

TIME
LIFE
BOOKS ®

HUMAN BEHAVIOR

the role of the brain

BY RONALD H. BAILEY

AND THE EDITORS OF TIME-LIFE BOOKS

TIME-LIFE BOOKS, NEW YORK

The Author: Ronald H. Bailey is a freelance author and journalist, formerly a senior editor of LIFE. He has published several articles on prison reform for the magazine *Corrections* and was a contributor to *The Unknown Leonardo,* a book about the inventive genius of Leonardo da Vinci. He and his wife and four children live on a farm in New York State.

General Consultants for Human Behavior:
Robert M. Krauss is Professor of Psychology at Columbia University. He has taught at Princeton and Harvard and was Chairman of the Psychology Department at Rutgers. He is the co-author of *Theories in Social Psychology,* edits the *Journal of Experimental Social Psychology* and contributes articles to many journals on aspects of human behavior and social interaction.

Peter I. Rose, a specialist on racial and ethnic relations, is Sophia Smith Professor of Sociology and Anthropology at Smith College and is on the graduate faculty of the University of Massachusetts. His books include *They and We, The Subject Is Race* and *Americans from Africa.* Professor Rose has also taught at Goucher, Wesleyan, Colorado, Clark, Yale, Amherst, the University of Leicester in England, Kyoto University in Japan and Flinders University in Australia.

James W. Fernandez is Chairman of the Anthropology Department at Dartmouth College. His research in culture change has taken him to East, West and South Africa and the Iberian peninsula. Articles on his field studies have been widely published in European and American anthropology journals. He has been president of the Northeastern Anthropological Association and a consultant to the Foreign Service Institute.

Special Consultant for The Role of the Brain:
Mitchell Glickstein is Professor of Psychology at Brown University and a member of the American Association of Anatomists, the American Physiological Society and an Associate Member of the British Physiological Society. He has published articles about the brain and behavior in the *Journal of Comparative Neurology,* the *Journal of Neurophysiology* and the *Journal of Comparative and Physiological Psychology.*

HUMAN BEHAVIOR
Editorial Staff for *The Role of the Brain:*
EDITOR: William K. Goolrick
Assistant Editor: Carole Kismaric
Text Editor: Betsy Frankel
Picture Editor: Sheila Osmundsen
Designer: John Martinez
Assistant Designers: Marion Flynn, Robert McKee
Staff Writers: Alice Kantor, Suzanne Seixas
Chief Researcher: Barbara Ensrud
Researchers: Oscar C. K. Chiang, Barbara Fleming,
Dunstan Harris, Ruth Kelton, Gail Nussbaum,
Robin Richman, Fred Ritchin, Heidi Sanford

Editorial Production
Production Editor: Douglas B. Graham
Assistant Production Editors: Gennaro C. Esposito,
Feliciano Madrid
Quality Director: Robert L. Young
Assistant Quality Director: James J. Cox
Copy Staff: Eleanore W. Karsten (chief),
Charles Blackwell, Susan B. Galloway,
Georgia Ingersoll, Florence Keith, Pearl Sverdlin
Picture Department: Dolores A. Littles
Martin Baldessari
Traffic: Carmen McLellan

Valuable assistance was given by the following
departments and individuals of Time Inc.: Editorial
Production, Norman Airey; Library, Benjamin
Lightman; Picture Collection, Doris O'Neil;
Photographic Laboratory, George Karas; TIME-LIFE
News Service, Murray J. Gart; Correspondents Ann
Natanson (Rome), Margot Hapgood and Dorothy
Bacon (London), Maria Vincenza Aloisi (Paris),
Elisabeth Kraemer (Bonn), Mary Johnson
(Stockholm), Lance Keyworth (Helsinki).

Contents

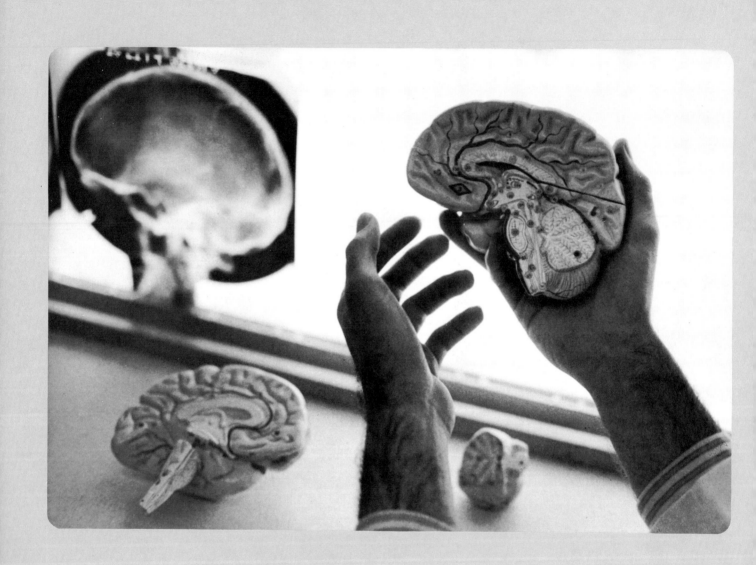

Geography of the Brain

1

As you sit quietly reading these words, the matter inside your skull bustles with activity. Millions of electrical currents so tiny that the sum of them could not illuminate an ordinary light bulb are flashing to and fro, performing small miracles you are scarcely aware of. They guide your eyes along the printed line, register the shapes of letters and, by matching the forms against memory, render them into words. They keep your heart beating, your lungs pumping. They monitor the feel of your hands upon this book and stand ready to order your fingers to turn the page. They may hear a noise in the other room, smell supper cooking or nag you about a disagreeable task left undone.

Most extraordinary of all, these unfelt activities inside your head tell you that you are reading about them; they make you aware of their unseen, unfelt presence and make it possible for you to contemplate the wonders of the human brain.

Perhaps more than any superlative, this image of the brain contemplating the brain brings home a truth that is often neglected in the observation of human behavior. Every thought, feeling or action begins in the brain and yet this fact is seldom given a thought. Instead, the coin of everyday speech is spent on other organs of the body. A surgeon's deftness is credited to his hands, a soldier's courage to his heart and certain intellectual qualities to a mysterious entity known as the mind. None of these, of course, is really responsible for human actions. It is the brain that is behavior's command post.

Only now are the astonishing quirks of brain operation beginning to be understood as scientists find explanations for such oddities of behavior as these:

☐ It is almost impossible to balance a pencil on the right forefinger and speak at the same time; the left forefinger does it much easier.

☐ Pricking the back of the hand with a pencil point may give a sensation of cold, not of pricking.

☐ Pressing one of the fingers against an eyelid does not stimulate a sensation of pressure alone but also makes the brain see a flash of light. □ No one can hold his breath more than about four minutes; after that he starts breathing whether he wants to or not.

□ Some boys seem to be born with girls' brains, and they act like girls while looking like boys.

The human brain is the most complex clump of matter known to man. Inside multiple layers of protection—the heavy thick bones of the skull, several membranes and a shock-absorbing cushion of fluid—lies the pinkish gray, wrinkled pudding that keeps a man alive. A bit larger than a grapefruit and weighing an average three and a half pounds, it looks like an overblown walnut. Incredibly sensitive to internal and external events, it is itself totally insensitive; the brain feels no pain directly, and surgeons are therefore able to work on it without using any anesthesia other than a local painkiller to deaden skin areas of the skull for incisions.

This remarkable organ is a conglomeration of several types of cells but it functions mainly with nerve cells. They are basically no different from the other nerve cells found throughout the body. Some of the body's nerves serve only as communications links. A large group runs from the brain in the main cable of the spinal cord, the foot-and-a-half-long bundle of nerves that extends down the back, then branches out to web the rest of the body. Some meet the muscles and control movement; others connect with sense organs such as the eyes and ears, where they pick up and send back to the brain various kinds of information about the body and the world around it.

All these nerves are similar in structure, although some are much larger than others. All operate in the same way. They generate energy from oxygen and sugar in the blood. Then they use this energy to send electrical signals from one cell to another—to make the fingers draw a picture, to actuate the mouth to say "I love you" or to inspire the mind to compose a sonnet. And yet despite physical similarities, these nerve cells are not all the same. Only the ones that are located in the retina of the eye respond to light, for example. Yet they do not see. Their responses must be relayed to other nerve cells in the brain, and only these cells—which themselves are insensitive to light—can convert the retinal response into an image.

Even in the brain, the nerve cells are not identical. They vary in size and shape and even more in function. Some are specialized—remove one small area behind the forehead and the capacity for anger may be eliminated, permanently. Other brain nerve cells are versatile, serving general purposes or taking over, when necessary, the tasks different

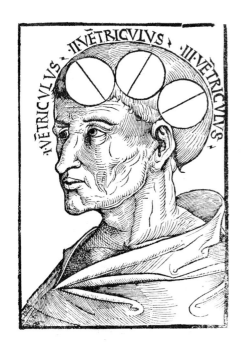

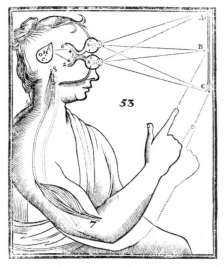

The 15th Century German philosopher Albertus Magnus believed that the brain's functions were housed in three bisected ventricles, as depicted in the woodcut at top. But the 17th Century French philosopher René Descartes believed that the brain's most important component was the pear-shaped pineal gland (at far left in lower drawing), which, he said, served as the home of the soul, receiver of visual stimuli and controller of muscular movements.

cells ordinarily perform. Altogether, the great, often mysterious, powers of the cells are what make human beings human.

A brain is not unique to man, of course. Even such a primitive creature as the half-inch-long flatworm possesses something at the head end of the body crudely approximating a brain.

But in man the elaboration of the brain took a decisive turn. Out of its maze of wrinkled gray matter arose the gift of language. Language enabled early man to communicate what he learned. His experience, stored in the brain as memory, could now be passed down from generation to generation. And a new kind of evolution took over, controlled by the human brain. With it man created the great edifice of civilization, vastly extending his cerebral gifts: machines to supplement his sensory and motor capabilities; housing to augment his built-in temperature mechanisms; taboos and laws to control instinctive emotions and drives; books and computers to aid memory.

Less successfully, man has sought to understand the mechanisms of his own behavior. Only in the last 300 years or so has it become clear that the brain alone is the physical source of behavior. And only in the last century have scientists begun systematically to map the many parts of the brain and relate them to specific activities. Today, this urgent task of learning why people act the way they do has become science's greatest challenge, the newest frontier. It has attracted many of the best minds from traditionally separate branches of study—biochemistry, psychology, anatomy, physiology and physics—and brought them together in an unprecedented assault upon the mystery of the human brain.

For many centuries most men were certain that the seat of behavior was not the brain at all but some other part of the body. The heart was most often singled out as the principal mechanism of human activity. It was a logical choice, for it could be felt pulsing with life; the tissue inside the head was silent. The Greek philosopher Plato parceled out behavior among three different parts of the body—attributing courage and ambition to the heart, reason to the head and baser qualities, such as desire and hunger, to the stomach. Aristotle felt sure the brain could not be the source of feelings because brain tissue is insensitive to pain. He suggested that the brain served merely as a radiator to cool the blood. But even long ago some inkling of the truth appeared. History's first recorded mention of the brain, in an Egyptian papyrus dating from 1700 B.C., shows some awareness that head wounds could result in lameness and blindness. And Hippocrates, the father of modern medicine, drew the correct conclusion from observations of patients who had suffered head injuries. He wrote: "Men ought to know that from the brain and from the brain only arise our pleasures, joys, laughter, and jests as well as our sorrows, pains, griefs and tears."

With the development of experimental science in the 16th and 17th centuries, the functions of the various organs of the body were learned and the importance of the brain understood. It came to be seen as a kind of living machine, subject to earthbound, discernible logic. If it is a kind of machine, then theoretically it can be broken down into parts. And each part might be tied to some observable act of behavior. This idea, known as localization and now a key doctrine in brain research, has become important only in the last century or so. Ironically, one of its early champions was the German anatomist Franz Joseph Gall, who is now considered something of a crank.

Gall believed a person's character could be analyzed by studying the bumps on his skull. He got this notion after he decided that the eyes of public speakers seemed to bulge. He then connected bulging eyes to the brain, maintaining that highly developed gray matter in the front of the brain pushed the eyes out. Gall and a cult of followers expanded his idea into a pseudo science, phrenology. They asserted that talents and temperament—everything from mathematical ability to cruelty—were distributed in distinct regions over the brain surface. If the skull bulged in a particular place, it was because the corresponding personality factor was expanding the gray matter.

Though Gall's reasoning was all wrong, part of his theory was right. Separate regions of the brain do relate directly to distinct aspects of behavior. In the 1860s, the French surgeon Paul Broca, conducting autopsies on patients with speech disorders, noticed that many of their brains were damaged in the same place; he thus located the region that controls speech. Then a pair of German physicians performed a key experiment using dogs. Eduard Hitzig had noted, while he was serving in the Prussian-Danish War, that soldiers with head wounds twitched their muscles if their brains were accidentally touched during treatment. He and Gustav Fritsch, working at home on Frau Hitzig's dressing table, inserted electric wires into the brain of a dog and found the area that controls voluntary movements. A burst of current in one place moved the dog's limbs; in a nearby place, it twitched the muscles of the head.

Today, 100 years of exploration have mapped in detail many behavioral areas of the brain. With these maps as a guide, it is possible to take an imaginary tour through the cerebral universe.

The tour begins at the base of the skull. Here the brain stem rises stalklike into the cranium from the top of the spinal cord. In the brain stem are two structures that together control the most primitive and essential

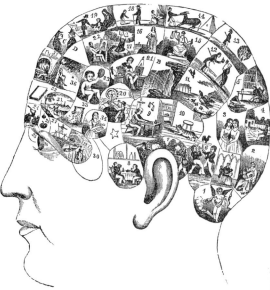

A phrenological chart links different areas of the skull with an assortment of personality traits and symbols—a nebulous quality called sublimity is represented by a waterfall at center (B). As befit the Victorian order of things, love of God resides at the highest level of the brain (18), while physical love is indicated by a coy Cupid (1) at the base.

A 19th Century cartoon satirizes the excitement with which fond parents rushed to have phrenologists "feel the bumps" on the heads of their babies.

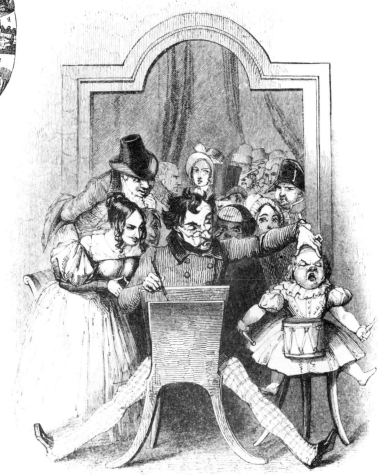

False clues from cranial bumps

During the 1800s, a pseudo science called phrenology swept Europe and America. Its founder, a Viennese doctor named Franz Gall, started with the sound idea that specific areas of the brain have specific capacities and functions. He added the incorrect notion that a protuberance on the skull indicated a well-developed brain area just beneath it. And from there he went on to the absurdity of ascribing specific traits and powers to the areas according to his own intuition.

His theories caught on. Thousands flocked to phrenological quacks, who surveyed skulls for everything from the ability to tell time to "amativeness" (the capacity for love). Queen Victoria sent her children to phrenologists and Karl Marx believed in phrenology.

By the 1850s the craze was fading, killed by its own preposterous claims just as surgeons like the Frenchmen Marc Dax and Paul Broca began to draw the true map of the areas and functions of the brain.

behavior, breathing itself. One is the medulla, near the lower part of the stem. The other is an arching area that must have looked like a hump-backed bridge to the anatomist who called it the pons—Latin for bridge. These two structures are connected by nerves to the chest muscles that expand and contract the lungs. Like other nerve connections between the brain and the body's trunk, the nerves travel via the spinal cord, the communications cable in the spinal column. A broken neck is so often fatal (and the hangman's noose therefore is efficient) because it can sever these nerves and stop respiration.

Breathing is a prime example of behavior that is prewired in the brain. It does not have to be learned, or even consciously willed, but continues semiautomatically. A person is often aware of his breathing, but he need not be—he breathes even while asleep. He can also control breathing, but only up to a point; if someone stops breathing for more than about four minutes, the automatic control takes over to start the lungs inhaling and to sustain the vital flow of oxygen.

The brain stem also contains other fundamental, semiautomatic systems such as the master switches of awareness—three different networks that regulate waking and sleep. One system, which extends from the stem to higher centers, arouses the brain like an alarm clock and alerts it to the importance of incoming information. It enables the brain to concentrate on first things first—for example, on the fact that the house is on fire—and to disregard all the other data streaming in from the senses. A second system switches on during sleep; a third system takes over during dreaming and makes certain the sleeper does not go through the physical motions of the dream. These parts of the brain apparently are most directly affected by drugs and by physical or mental efforts—rituals, meditation—that seek to alter states of consciousness.

Fore and aft of the brain stem, hanging from the stalk like tiny fruit, are two glands. They are not nerve tissue but they serve as the main regulators of body chemistry and so powerfully affect behavior that they are considered part of the brain. The pituitary, in front, secretes the chemical messengers called hormones, which influence a range of bodily functions and behavior, from growth to the female reproductive cycle. (Birth-control pills work their effects by acting upon the pituitary.) The pineal gland, in back of the stem, was called the seat of the soul by the 17th Century philosopher René Descartes. Its actual functions appear to have more to do with sex. It secretes hormones involved in the development of sexual organs and acts as a biological clock, a built-in timekeeper, for the menstrual cycle.

Perched on the highest rear branch of the brain stem is a much larger structure, the plum-sized cerebellum, the "lesser brain." It maintains the body's equilibrium and coordinates muscles during fine movements —for example, it enables the fingers to thread a needle without overshooting the mark.

The brain stem and its associated structures are practically hidden by two connected bodies that arch above and around them, the cerebral hemispheres. At the core of the hemispheres is the thalamus, the central switchboard between the spinal cord and the brain's upper levels. All sensations pass through here except smell, which has its own private connection to the higher centers, an inch-long olfactory bulb that juts forward from the base of each cerebral hemisphere and carries the news from the nose directly to the brain. This main-line connection, which is unique among the body's senses, may explain the extraordinary ability of odors—perfume, the smell of cooking—to evoke some of the most powerful of human memories.

Below the thalamus lies a tiny but complex center of emotions and drives, the hypothalamus. It sets off instinctive behavior aimed at self preservation. It warns of hunger and thirst. It triggers sexual activities. It commands the body's responses to stress—quickened heartbeat, fluttery stomach, cold hands. Most dramatically, it generates intense feelings of anger, fear and even pleasure.

The hypothalamus appears to work in tandem with a series of related deep-seated emotional controls, known collectively as the limbic system. The limbic system forms a kind of ring in each of the cerebral hemispheres. One part of this system, the hippocampus (from the Greek for sea horse), is believed essential for the formation and storage of new memories.

Above the limbic system, in the crumpled covering of the cerebral hemispheres, is the cortex, where man's special gifts reside. Here, among densely packed mats of nerve cells, are the centers responsible for the uniqueness of human behavior: the capacity for language, the delicate motor control that makes possible the use of tools, the safety devices that manage built-in drives and emotions, the interpretive systems that enable man to perceive himself and the world around him. Birds have almost no cortex at all, and the derisive term "birdbrain" is consequently highly appropriate. Mammals such as rats have a cortex but it is smooth. The human cortex has grown so large that, stretched out flat, it would form a sheet about an eighth of an inch thick, a yard long and two feet wide. In order to fit within the confines of the skull, it folds in upon itself —a trick that triples the surface area.

The cortical folds create a rugged topography of ridges and furrows. Several of the furrows are so deep they serve as identifying features on the cortical terrain, demarcating each hemisphere into four separate regions, or lobes. Each of these lobes takes its name from a nearby bone in the skull.

The occipital lobe, at the back of the head, contains the visual cortex, which receives sensations of light from the eyes. Microscopic nerve cells here respond to the incoming data in a remarkably specific way—one cell responds only to one tiny bit of the image. Together the cells build up a kind of mental mosaic. This is the picture created by vision, perceived in the brain and not in the eyes.

The parietal lobe, at the top of the head, monitors the sensation of touch and keeps track of the location of the movable parts of the body. Scientists call this part of the brain the somesthetic area (from the Greek for body sensation) to differentiate it from regions concerned with other sensory impressions. Distinct points in it monitor the different parts of the body in inverted order—detectors for foot location are at the top of the lobe; those for the tongue near the bottom. This perception of the body is what enables a man to walk and run without tripping over his feet and to lower himself confidently into a chair. Its delicacy is developed to the most remarkable degree not in humans, however, but in mice and rats. Equipped with long, sensitive whiskers for feeling their way through walled habitats, they have correspondingly elaborate parietal lobes. The somesthetic area in these rodents contains a number of barrel-shaped structures, each of which is activated by a single whisker.

Just below the parietal lobe, at the side of the head by the temple, is the temporal lobe. It carries out advanced tasks: hearing and the understanding of language. Moreover, experiments with monkeys suggest that at least one type of memory may be stored in the temporal lobe —the kind that comes to the brain via vision.

Around in front, behind the forehead, the frontal lobe receives the sense of smell and performs two other functions. The back portion is the motor cortex, the command center for voluntary movement, divided according to bodily topography. The key speech center, not surprisingly, abuts the parts of the motor cortex that control jaw, tongue and other movements necessary for speech. It is also near the hand-control area—a hint that human ancestors may have communicated through hand signals. The remainder of the frontal lobe, the prow of gray matter overhanging the eyes, is a mystery, though many scientists believe it contains centers of intention or foresight that enable man to plan ahead.

If this tour of the brain seems to have left something out, the omis-

continued on page 18

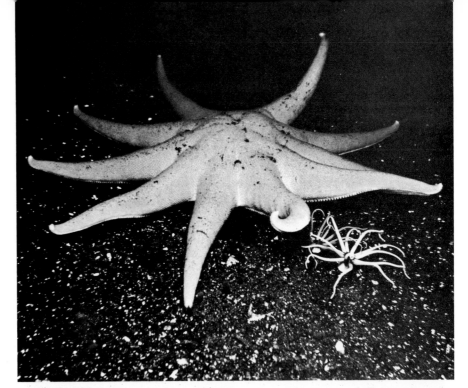

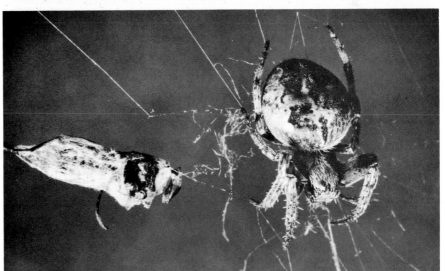

The starfish, an invertebrate ocean dweller, lacks a centralized brain. Nerve networks located on the underside of its body send sensations of touch directly to its muscles; movements are slow and quite poorly coordinated.

Using a high skill programed into a tiny brain, a spider wraps a paralyzed wasp into a silky cocoon for storage. The spider was alerted to its prey by fine body hairs, which sensed vibrations in the web.

Evolving toward man's mind

The brain is absolutely essential to human life. Yet oddly enough this exquisite mechanism is actually one of nature's happier afterthoughts.

A brain is not essential to every creature. Some have none, and others get along very well with crude ones. Insects, with the most rudimentary of brains, swarmed over the earth millions of years before man and now outnumber him millions of times over. But the size and complexity of a brain does tell something about its owner's place in evolution: the earlier the appearance of any type of animal on the earth, the more primitive its brain.

The early animals, such as the starfish (*top*) lacked brains. Later arrivals, such as the spider (*above*), had only a clump of nerve connections at one end of the body. Still later came the reptiles with complete but small brains; some of them were 10-ton monsters with brains the size of a kitten's. Only in the mammals, the most recent of the major animal groups, did the brain attain the size and richness needed for emotion and intelligence.

These crocodiles, basking in a Florida stream, possess in their brains every element of the human brain—even the cerebrum, center of thought. But the crocodile is guided by instinct, not thought; its cerebrum is mainly concerned with taste and smell.

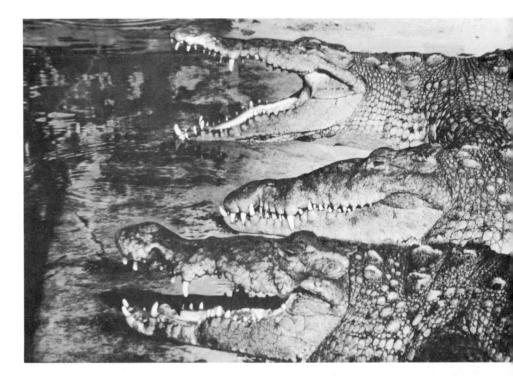

Like almost all mammals, elephants have large, highly developed brains. Indeed, their brains are huge, weighing an average of 13 pounds. But that size is deceptive. For every pound of brain, an elephant has almost a thousand pounds of body (the human ratio is 1 to 50) so most of the elephant brain is devoted to coordinating its massive bulk.

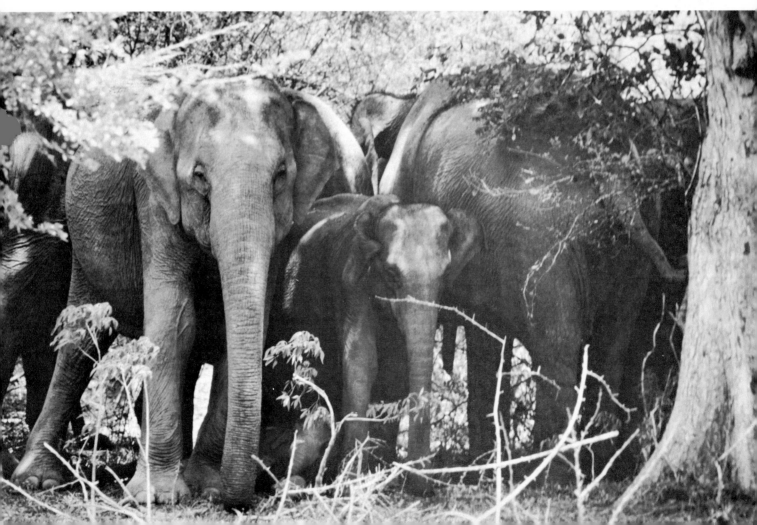

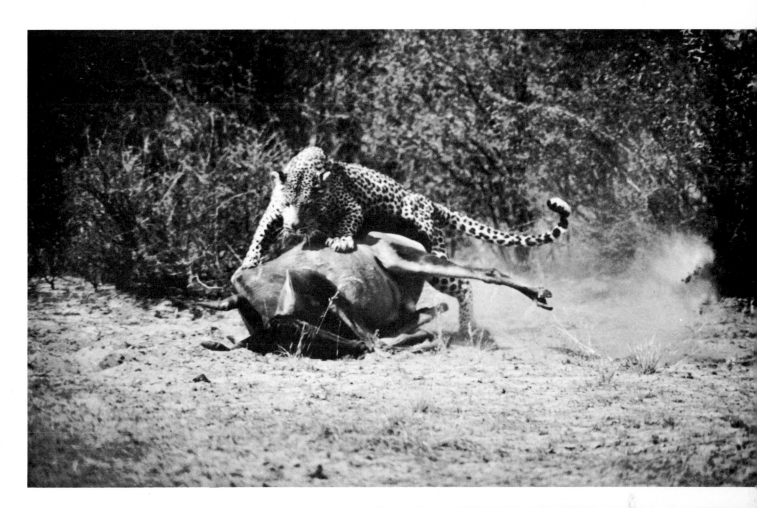

The leopard has to move and think faster
than the elephant to catch a meal like the
antelope above. Hunting cats have brains
(and bodies) designed for split-second
timing and lightning coordination—and
for the long attention span needed to stalk
their prey for hours on end.

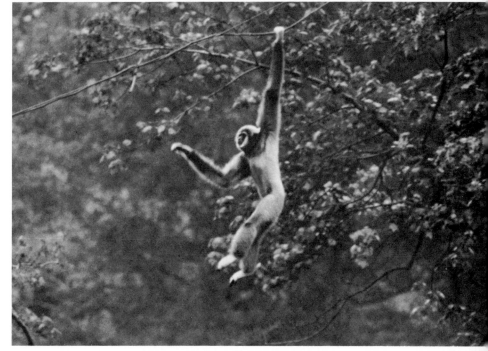

Swinging gracefully through an African
forest, a gibbon makes use of a brain that
approaches the brain of a man in
complexity. Like man, the gibbon enjoys
stereoscopic vision and fine muscle
coordination. More significantly, it judges
situations with a cerebrum capable of
extensive learning and thought.

sion is unavoidable. Three fourths of the cortical terrain is uncharted. Somewhere in these labyrinths reside the most important and enigmatic of man's attributes—thought, creativity, love.

The century-long effort to map the brain and determine which nerve cells control which activity has established a striking and significant characteristic of its structures: like most parts of the body, the elements that constitute the brain come in pairs. Just as there are two lungs and paired limbs, there are two cerebellums and two cerebral hemispheres. In terms of behavior, brain and body together can be regarded as split vertically down the middle, with half of the brain relating to half of the body. For some unknown reason, however, the nerves from the body perversely cross over in the spinal cord going to and from the brain. The effect of this crossing is that each side of the brain presides over the opposite side of the body.

The mirror-like functioning of brain parts reveals itself dramatically in the disorder known as parietal lobe syndrome, in which one of the two halves of the lobe is affected. The brain area involved monitors touch and body awareness, but only on one side of the body—if the right half of the lobe suffers, awareness of the left side of the body is lost. The victim, lacking reports from an entire half of his body, tends to forget it is there and neglects it. Often, he presents the image of a split person—half well groomed, half unkempt. In one case a patient's leg seemed so alien to him that he shot it because he thought it belonged to an intruder in his home; the failure of perception led him in a rational way to an irrational act.

Though the sensory centers in each cerebral hemisphere are essentially mirror twins, the hemispheres are not the same. One hemisphere generally determines which hand will be used for delicate tasks like writing; most people are right-handed, which means that control of this function usually comes from the left hemisphere. More remarkable, the capacity for speech and language generally resides in one hemisphere. In 97 out of 100 persons, it is the left hemisphere. This concentration of verbal ability on one side of the brain is what makes it so difficult to talk while balancing a pencil on the index finger of the right hand. The two simultaneous acts, speaking and controlling fine digital movement, put a double burden on the left hemisphere. It is less difficult if the balancing act is performed with the left hand.

The left hemisphere's control over language often becomes evident in cases of stroke, caused by a blocked blood vessel. The blockage may cut off the oxygen supply to any of several language centers on the left side, killing clusters of delicate nerve cells. A brain specialist often can

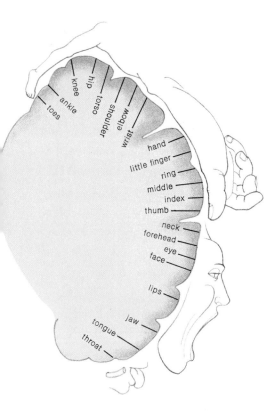

If the human body were proportioned the way the brain's muscle-operating circuits are, the hand would be its biggest part with the mouth and tongue (needed for speech) close behind; the legs and torso would be comparatively small. The sketches above, relating body size to motor areas in the brain, are adapted from the concept of Canadian neurosurgeon Wilder Penfield, a pioneer in exploration of the human brain.

predict the site of damage from the symptoms of the language impairment. If the patient speaks with great difficulty in a telegraphic style that omits endings of verbs and nouns, the damage has hurt an area near the motor cortex of the left hemisphere. If roundabout phrases are substituted for a simple word—"What you use to cut with" instead of "knife"—the area affected may be the language center in the left temporal lobe. The inability to comprehend written language implicates an area in the left part of the brain, one that is directly connected to the visual area.

In recent years an extraordinary series of experiments has shown that the specialization of each hemisphere extends beyond language and hand use. In most people the left hemisphere controls not only language but other abilities of a logical nature such as mathematics, while the right hemisphere has special artistic talents. The fact that all normal human brains work much alike, the same section in each controlling the same activities, is something of a surprise.

Behavior is so infinitely varied that brains might be expected to come in a variety of structures, sizes and shapes. They do not. Except for some dependence on body weight—women's brains average a scant 10 per cent smaller than men's because women weigh less—all brains are much alike in form and chemical makeup. The brains of notable individuals—Einstein, Lenin, Napoleon—have been examined with great interest after death, and they did not appear to be much different from anyone else's. The basic physical similarity reflects specificity of the brain—the precision with which evolution laid down cerebral wiring patterns and established their development.

The growth of an individual's brain follows a set schedule from the time he is conceived. A few days after conception, the brain consists of a straight smooth tube too small to be seen without a microscope. In the next nine months the tube will reenact, in a rough way, 300 million years of evolution. At various stages, it will superficially resemble the brains of creatures lower on the evolutionary ladder—ascending from fish to reptile to mammal.

In the seventh week, the tube sprouts three bumps and begins to take shape. At one end the tube will extend to become the spinal cord, the communications cable common to fish and all other creatures with a backbone. The two bumps nearest that end will become the brain stem and acquire structures responsible for such primitive reflexes as breathing and heartbeat. The third bump will first produce centers for emotions and drives (which were dominant in man's reptilian ancestors 100 million years ago) and then sprout above and around them the huge cerebral hemispheres. The behavior of the unborn baby follows the refinement of the three bumps. By three weeks his own nervous system, not his mother's, controls his heartbeat. By 12 weeks he kicks when his mother presses her abdomen.

Shortly before birth, a mysterious event with momentous impact on future behavior occurs in the womb. The sex of the embryonic brain is fixed. Animal experiments indicate that no matter which set of genital organs have developed in the body—whether the embryo is physically male or female—the brain's wired-in pattern of sexual behavior is female. At this point, long after the genes and sex hormones have dictated a male body, additional sex hormones must act upon the brain and make it male. If they do not, the embryo will develop a female brain in a male body—and the boy will grow up to act feminine.

At birth the human baby's brain already possesses its full complement of electricity-conducting nerve cells. (In the womb they have proliferated at the astounding rate of 20,000 per minute.) But as the baby's elementary behavior makes clear, the brain is far from complete. The baby sucks, cries, thrashes his limbs; most of this is the work of innate reflexes controlled by the brain's lower regions, which are almost in full operating condition at the time of birth. Motor areas controlling movements of the upper body are somewhat developed but sensory areas lag behind. The infant can see at birth, but he apparently discerns only the sensations of light and dark. He is not yet ready to appreciate the outside world because his cortex, the upper brain layer that interprets and thinks, is relatively undeveloped. It requires longer to mature in humans than in any other creature.

During the first two years of life, the brain and consequent behavior change with extraordinary speed. Two occurrences make possible the baby's rapid acquisition of new skills. The nerves send out numerous branching fibers, which connect with other fibers to complete new behavioral circuits. At the same time, cells within the nerves proliferate, enabling them to transmit signals more speedily.

Partly as a result of these two developments, the weight of the infant brain doubles during the first six months of life.

By the third month, the baby controls many conscious movements. He begins to grasp objects with his hands and to coordinate this action by using his eyes, focusing on an object and reaching for it. Soon the hearing area of the brain enables him to recognize the sound of his mother's voice and he stops crying when she soothes him. By seven months, the muscle-control sections of the upper cortex empower him to crawl, by the ninth month to stand, by the 12th month to walk. Thereafter lan-

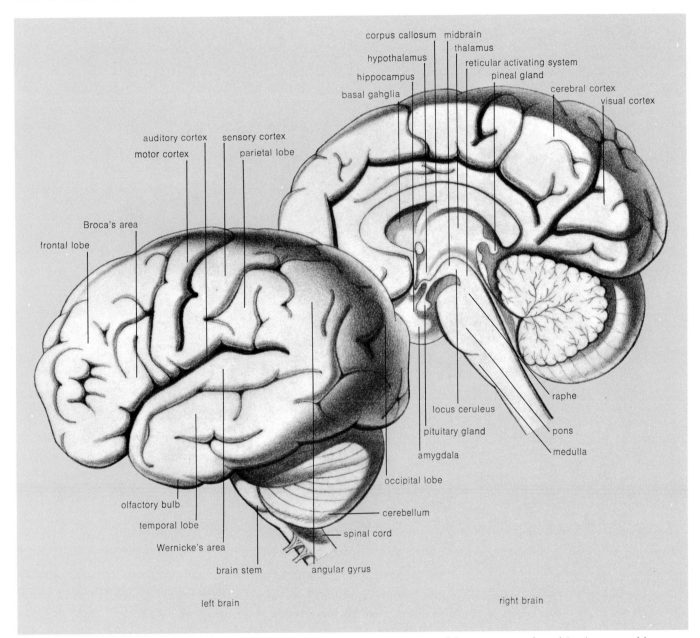

corpus callosum · midbrain
hypothalamus · thalamus
hippocampus · reticular activating system
basal ganglia · pineal gland
cerebral cortex
visual cortex

auditory cortex · sensory cortex
motor cortex · parietal lobe

Broca's area
frontal lobe

locus ceruleus
pituitary gland
amygdala
occipital lobe
cerebellum
spinal cord
raphe
pons
medulla

olfactory bulb
temporal lobe
Wernicke's area
brain stem · angular gyrus

left brain   right brain

Split down the middle to show interior and exterior features, the brain is illustrated here as a complex of intricate, sensitive parts.

The architecture of the brain

The many parts of the brain that govern behavior fit into two halves identical in structure but not in function, —in effect, two separate brains. The most prominent feature is the domed cerebrum, whose wrinkled surface, the cerebral cortex, contains controls for senses and muscles. Deep fissures divide the cerebral cortex into four lobes—

frontal, temporal, parietal and occipital.

The brain's other main parts are the cerebellum, a coordinator of muscles, and the brain stem, which contains mechanisms to control alertness.

In this split view of the brain, some components are located by general areas. More specific locations are delineated on pages 30 to 43.

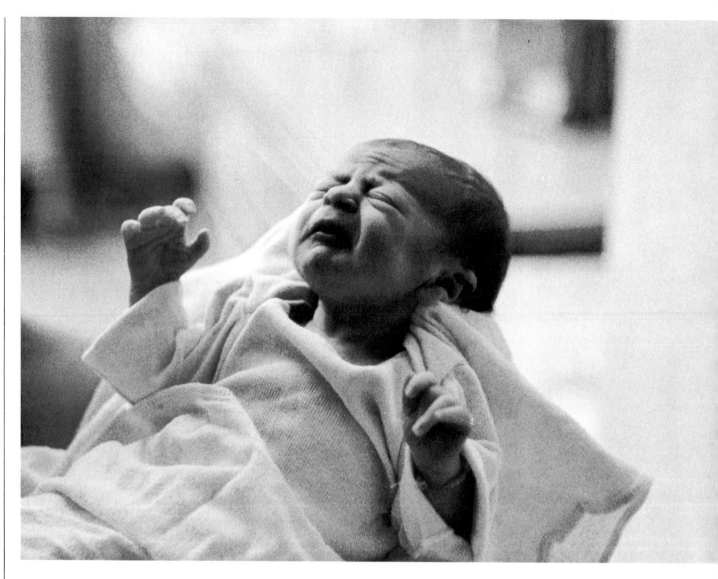

guage areas develop to produce speech and, in ways that still remain mysterious, the in-between areas that permit the association of ideas combine to yield the wonders of human personality.

This time schedule occasionally is subject to interruption because of the developing brain's high vulnerability to disease and injury. Inherited defects, built into the genes bequeathed a baby by his parents, may result in a lack of brain chemicals essential to normal intelligence, dooming the child, before birth, to mental retardation. Or they may bring about blockage of the fluid that helps cushion and nourish the brain. Such a blockage can enlarge the cavernous spaces, called ventricles, that supply blood to the brain cells, swelling the head so grotesquely that the victim of this affliction is said to have "water on the brain"—technically, hydrocephalus.

A human baby is far more helpless than other newborn animals because his brain, unlike theirs, is immature at birth. In the newborn baby at left, only the brain stem —the area controlling such involuntary actions as breathing, kicking and crying —is operational. Over the next six months, however, growth in the areas that control voluntary movement and thinking will double the weight of his brain.

Birth itself presents a peril. Most babies are delivered head first, and the infant brain is unusually large—about one fifth of body weight. It is easily hurt as the head is squeezed, and sometimes pulled by instruments, through the mother's narrow pelvic opening. Though the brain is protected by the skull, three outer layers of membrane and a fluid cushion, a blow can damage an entire section of tissue. Another hazard during birth is lack of oxygen. The demands of the infant's brain are huge, taking as much as 50 per cent of the available supply. Oxygen deficiency or a blow to the head is a cause of cerebral palsy, a tragically common disorder in which damage to the brain cells prevents the normal development of essential functions—bodily movements, speech and intellectual abilities *(pages 66-77)*.

The development of the brain does not stop with birth, of course. Simply bouncing and jiggling a baby can be dangerous, according to a Pittsburgh pediatrician, John Caffey. The infant's heavy but weakly supported head may be flopped back and forth so hard that brain blood vessels bleed, leading to the formation of membranes that interfere with brain growth. Caffey speculates that shaking young children may cause mental retardation. "Many slow-learning and clumsy children with IQ's of 90" he says, "might have been intelligent and normally mobile children with IQ's of 120, had they not been habitually shaken and whiplashed during infancy."

Even the paint on a baby's crib may threaten the growing brain. Eating flakes of paint that contain lead causes brain cells to swell, and the effect on behavior can be catastrophic: severe mental retardation or death. If eating the wrong things can harm the behavior control centers, so too may not eating enough of the right things. Malnutrition, many experiments have shown, stunts mental development in animals. The evidence for similar effects on humans is less direct and far from certain but persuasive to some experts. Field studies in Latin America indicate that mental development lags in ill-fed children. These observations suggest that malnutrition in infants (or in their mothers before they are born) may result in smaller head size—and presumably a smaller brain. Worse, the animal experiments imply that the behavioral influence of malnutrition in the mother may be visited not only upon her children but upon her grandchildren—even if the offspring themselves receive an adequate diet.

Subtler yet—and more debatable—are the effects on the brain of experience. Evidence from animal studies shows some measurable changes from experience and helps illuminate, but by no means resolve, the old argument: Is behavior shaped more by heredity or environment? Experiments involving the visual system, for example, suggest that there are crucial times during development when the brain must interact with the environment. If infant kittens are deprived of vision at the wrong time, by having their eyes temporarily kept shut, they lose the use of certain pathways in the brain and go blind. In young chicks an important event, which is known to change the brain chemically, occurs during the first 24 hours of life. The chicks' eyes imprint upon their brains an image that thereafter becomes something they consider their "mother" —even if the image is not their real mother but no more than a series of flashing lights or the scientist himself.

More interesting environmental effects on the brain have been reported in experiments with rats at the University of California. Litter mates were divided into two groups after weaning: in one group each rat was reared alone in a cage empty of things to play with or to invite attention; the rats in the other group were raised in a communal cage luxuriously outfitted with ladders, trapezes and other challenging diversions. The brains of the rats raised in the enriched environment changed chemically, the investigators reported, and developed thicker, heavier cortices. These differences presumably made the rats raised in the stimulating environment smarter than those in the unstimulated group. These findings have been seized upon by proponents of early childhood education, who say the experiments prove the value of enriching the experiences of humans at a very young age. Most experts, however, are cautious about drawing such conclusions.

Whatever the significance for human behavior of animal tests, there can be no doubt that any human experience—playing with toys, meeting people, reading books, listening to music—leaves some imprint on the brain. If the experience is remembered at all (and only in rare circumstances is it totally, irrevocably forgotten), then a tangible change in the physical makeup of the brain has taken place. It may be the production of some specific chemical—a "memory molecule"—or, more likely, the establishment of specific patterns in the complex connections between brain cells. At any time, this physical trace of experience can influence behavior, connecting a name to a face or bringing into play a seemingly unknown skill.

The imprint of experience gets to the brain by way of the sense organs, which, like the brain, are made of nerve cells. Although they are not part of the brain, they are connected to it—necessarily so. For the brain's very awareness of the body and the outside world depends upon the constant stream of information flowing in from the senses. The senses are the crucial go-betweens, the elaborately contrived mechanisms

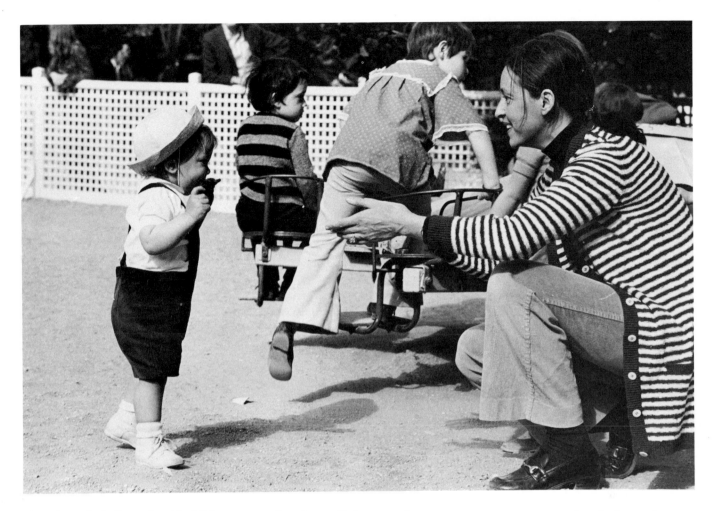

At twelve and a half months, this child takes his first hesitant steps. During the previous year, the motor cortex and cerebellum areas of his brain, involved in muscle control, have been growing steadily; now, beginning his second year of life, he has acquired the myelin nerve sheaths (page 48) that help him to be able to walk and speak.

that detect light, sound, pressure, temperature or chemicals, and translate this news into simple electrical impulses.

The eyes, ears and other sensory outposts send 100 million separate coded messages to the brain every second. These messages are the raw materials of awareness, the unprocessed input. How the brain processes raw sensations, interpreting them in the light of mood, expectations and other variables, is known as perception. A familiar illustration of the distinction between sensation and perception is pain. The same sensation —the signals from a cavity in a tooth, for example—affects each person differently. His suffering is the perception. It varies with the individual brain's response to the sensation.

Senses, like the brain, have evolved with man, adapting to provide new behavior suited to new conditions. Smell, a key sense in lower mammals such as dogs, became less important when some ancient primate —ancestor to monkeys, apes and humans—moved from the ground to trees. Sight had a better potential for the instantaneous reporting necessary to clutch at branches and clamber safely through the perilous

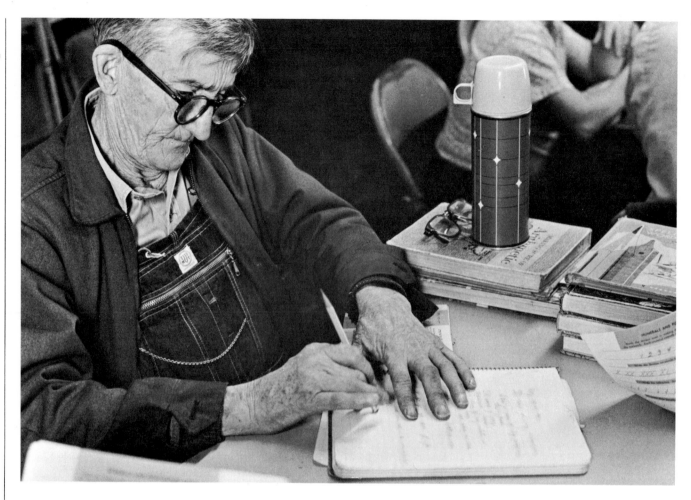

heights. The eyes developed millions of additional cells responsive to light and moved from the side of the head to the front. Their new location made the sensations from each eye overlap in the brain in just the right way to provide binocular vision, the three-dimensional view that improves the judgment of depth.

The evolution of speech some 100,000 years ago also involved significant physical changes. It depended on refinements in hearing. Human ears became complex gadgets, each an unlikely combination of tiny bones, membranes, fluids and 50,000 cells equipped with fine hairs that pluck vibrations of sound from the air. Meanwhile, taste was downgraded by evolution. Basically, a human can now distinguish only whether food is sweet, sour, salty or bitter. Much of the subtle power attributed to the 10,000 taste buds more properly belongs to touch, the arbiter of texture, and to the sense of smell (which is why a stopped-up nose leaves food largely tasteless).

The senses embedded in the skin—touch, temperature, pain—tend to cluster at those places that have proved significant in man's evolution. Man's tool-wielding hands are equipped with as many as 30 times more tiny nerve endings for touch than equivalent areas in less useful parts of the body. For the transmission of pain, the hands and some other areas have two different types of pain-sensitive nerve endings: one produces a reaction faster than the other. Quick response to pain is so obviously essential to survival that a "hot-stove" reflex has been built into the nervous system: the hand draws back from a painful burn automatically, without direct intervention from the brain. Only later does the second sensation get through to inform the brain that the stove was indeed dangerously hot.

The senses also have evolved as organs of limitation. Evolution has made them insensitive to anything not of practical use; thus they protect the brain from being overwhelmed with unneeded information. Human eyes, for example, detect only a narrow band of the spectrum —those colors most advantageous for sharp vision in daylight—and they are not sensitive to infrared, ultraviolet or X-rays. (But the brain magnifies sight enormously by enabling man to create electronic and photographic devices with which he can perceive these invisible rays when he wants to.)

Understanding the process by which the brain converts raw sensations into perception presents far more complications. Sensation varies only according to the power of the stimulus; perception varies by an infinity of factors within the brain itself. The result is that the brain is easily deceived by sensation.

Pressure on the eye is easily read as light. A more painful demonstration, a blow to the eye, makes the victim see stars. There is also a cold-sensitive nerve ending on the back of the hand that is stimulated by probing lightly with the point of a pencil. The stimulus is mechanical pressure, but the resulting message to the brain says "cold." At one point on the elbow, four different types of nerve endings are bundled together—touch, pain, heat and cold. A sharp blow there elicits a confusing mixture of sensations that is recorded by the brain as a painful and eerie tingling.

Subtler and more important confusion may arise when the brain must interpret a variety of sensations. Witnesses to an automobile accident take in essentially the same sensations; their accounts of what they have seen and heard always differ. Expectations, based on memory, enable optical illusions to trick the brain—such illusions are designed to evoke familiar but misleading patterns in the mind's eye. "What a piece of bread looks like," wrote a 13th Century Persian poet, "depends on whether you are hungry or not."

27

A modern experiment bears out the powerful influence that the individual's expectations have on perception: When a group of poor and rich children were shown certain coins, the poor ones tended to think the coins they saw were larger in size than did their more fortunate peers. The state of emotions also may have a decisive effect. As the mood dictates, a simple touch on the arm may be interpreted as a caress or a bother.

Even though the brain is often uncertain in its interpretation of sensations, the process of perception must follow some logical procedure in order, for example, that a stream of electrical impulses from the ears be perceived as a nightingale's song. Investigation of the visual system suggests a workable theory. In the brain's sensory areas, individual nerve cells serve as pattern detectors. These cells respond to nerve signals that arrive in a specific pattern; the signals are coded and transmitted to a nearby area of the brain's surface, where they are somehow composed into a coherent mosaic. (In vision, damage to this nearby area causes "mind blindness"—the victim can tell light from dark but cannot recognize patterns.) Finally, in remote reaches of the brain, a cell must serve as a comparing mechanism, matching the mosaic against the myriad patterns stored in the brain's memory in order to confirm that one particular sound pattern constitutes the nightingale's song and not that of the meadowlark.

It is easy to see why such a delicate, complex process as perception can so easily go awry accidentally—or be made to do so on purpose. There has been no dearth of deliberate tinkering for a variety of purposes. People with emotional disorders can often be helped by drugs that influence the way the brain interprets signals from the outside world. Tranquilizers, for example, alleviate irrational fears and worries, apparently by affecting the way signals move from one circuit to another within the brain. In some cases, surgeons have attempted to eradicate violent behavior, sexual deviance and lesser misconduct by burning out small bits of the brain.

Such radical intervention with the functions of the brain can backfire, however, for the distinct parts of the brain are not separate but work together in intricate and unknown ways. Tinkering with one part tends to affect another part, producing unpredictable behavior. One bank executive underwent a brain operation to relieve the severe pain of cancer. This aim was achieved, but there was a side effect (less serious than those suffered by many patients). After recovering from the operation he took his wife to the opera. Immaculate in formal evening attire, he walked with her to the theater and seemed his normal witty self.

Halfway there, however, he said "Excuse me" and, in full view of passersby, urinated in the street.

The reasons for interfering with the brain's processes of perception and interpretation are most often not medical, however. From the most ancient times, men have sought to change their perceptions of the world and of themselves, deliberately altering their thoughts in an effort to expand their sense of awareness. Generally the purpose is relatively trivial; people consume alcohol to relax and enjoy themselves. But there may also be a more serious goal. Art and literature, ritual and meditation, hallucinogenic drugs—all aim to change perceptions so that the mind can transcend the limitations of the earth-bound brain. "Our normal waking consciousness . . . is but one special type of consciousness," wrote the psychologist William James, "whilst all about it, parted from it by the filmiest of screens, there lie potential forms of consciousness entirely different."

James's words, written nearly a century ago, grew out of his hallucinogenic experience with nitrous oxide, the "laughing gas" that is used in anesthesia. In recent years, more potent mind drugs such as LSD have become the medium through which some people have sought to expand consciousness; others have turned for the same purpose to Eastern methods of meditation.

Such efforts to expand the mind imply a mysterious entity that somehow transcends the brain. Most people separate the concept of the mind from the pinkish gray tissue inside the head. The separation is institutionalized in sciences such as psychoanalysis, which seeks to understand man without reference to the physical reality of brain functions. But the existence of the mind as a thing apart from the brain is questionable.

Many scientists assert that the mind is merely "the ghost in the machine"—mind and brain are one and the same. They believe that the solutions to the mysteries of the mind will someday be found in the physical brain, amid the wiring of the enchanted machine that transforms electrical energy into the infinite variety of human behavior.

The master controls of behavior

Occupying the entire top of the human head is nature's most tantalizing, talented and versatile creation, the wrinkled, three and a half pound jellylike clump of the brain. In one way or another, it is the center of all behavior.

The brain is a filing system for millions of bits of information, a language center that sorts and arranges many thousands of words in an almost infinite variety of combinations. It is the constant monitor of a flood of sensory impressions from the outer world, the principal generator of human drives and emotions, and the operator of such vital functions as breathing *(right)*, heartbeat and muscle movements.

But what is most remarkable about the brain is that it can do all of these things and think at the same time. A man can be standing on a podium waving his arms and making a speech, and his brain will be figuring out what he ought to say next, calling up from his mental filing system the necessary ideas, regulating his body functions, controlling his muscles, forming phrases, and all the while registering the reactions of his audience.

For more than 150 years scientists have been probing the brain in an effort to find out what part of it does what when and why. They have been astonishingly successful. By conducting autopsies on the dead and by stimulating live subjects electrically, they have located the language and speech centers, mapped the motor and sensory control areas with precision, and pinpointed the control of respiration, alertness and sleep. Now scientists are tuning in on the activities of single cells within these circuits as, slowly and painstakingly, they continue to unravel the intriguing mystery of the human brain.

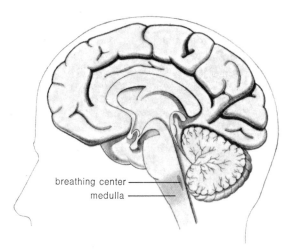

breathing center ———
medulla ———

A cross section of the brain shows vital respiratory centers in the lower part of the medulla, which control the rate and depth of breathing as well as the expansion and contraction of the chest.

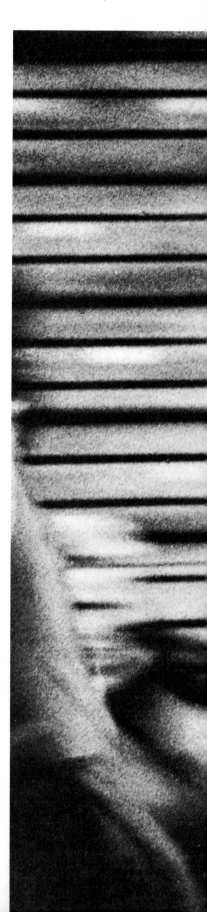

Straining to win a 100-meter sprint, Swedish runners gasp for breath during a Stockholm track-and-field meet. For each breath, the brain oversees the coordination of 90 muscles.

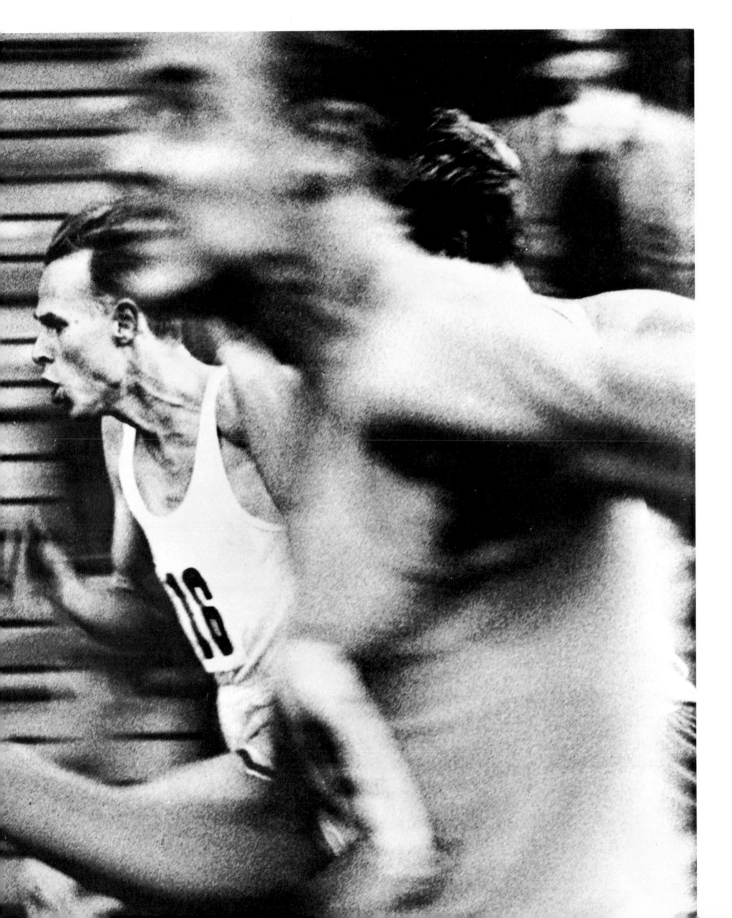

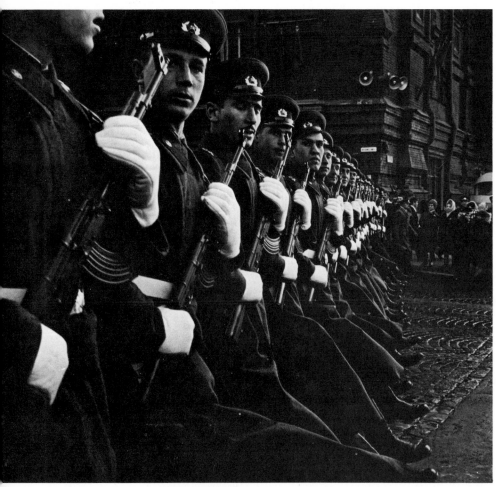

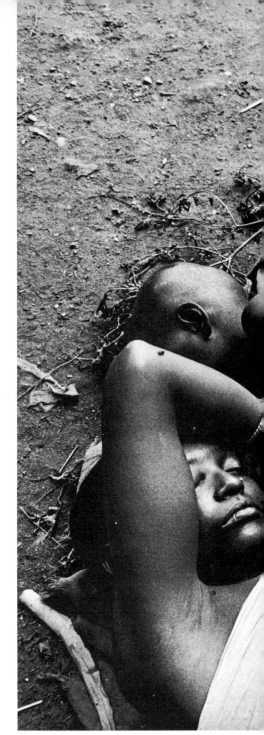

The RAS consciousness circuits in their brains set for alertness, Soviet soldiers try to keep movements and expressions coordinated as they march past the reviewing stand during a parade honoring the anniversary of the Revolution.

An exhausted mother and her three children renew their energies in sleep at a refugee camp during the 1971 war between India and Bangladesh. Sleep is apparently needed more for mental refreshment than for physical rest.

The reticular activating system, or RAS, located in the upper portion of the brain stem, governs both wakefulness and sleep. Alertness is controlled by RAS nerve fibers in the pons, while the centers that control deep and light sleep are located in the upper region of the RAS, which projects into the midbrain.

midbrain

reticular activating system

pons

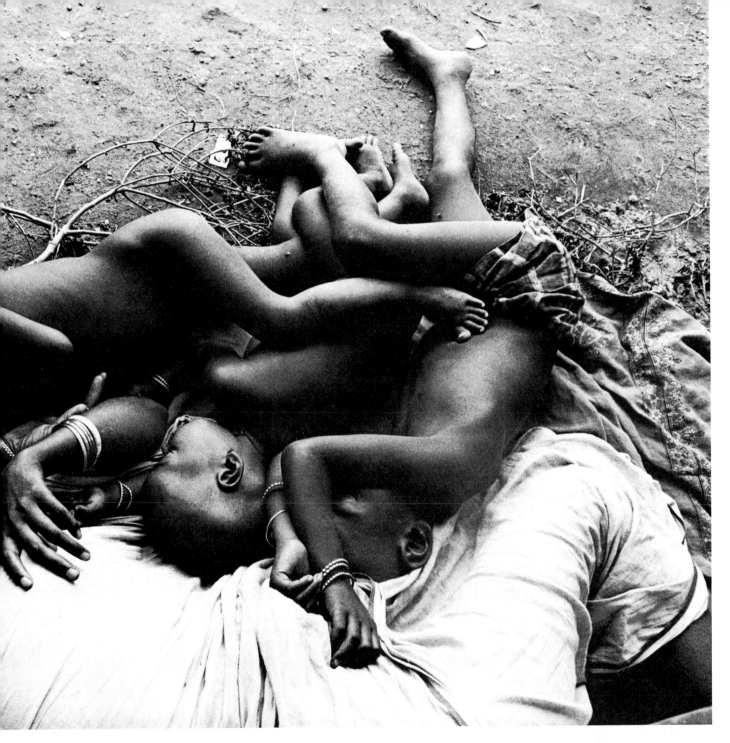

Switching levels of alertness

From a wide-awake alertness to day-dreaming, light sleep and deep sleep, the normal levels of human consciousness are regulated mainly by a two- to three-inch finger-shaped structure within the brain known as the reticular activating system, or RAS, which spans two trunk-line switching sections of the brain, the pons and midbrain. The RAS shifts in consciousness from one level to another are not always clearly seen in an individual's external behavior, but they can be pinpointed precisely from changes they cause in the rhythm of electrical currents the brain generates.

Experiments that involved electrical stimulation of cats have implicated the RAS in these brain-wave alterations and indicated the mechanism that alters consciousness. Apparently nerve fibers secrete chemicals—serotonin and norepinephrine—that stimulate or depress the RAS to switch awareness levels between deep sleep and alertness.

Mechanisms for survival

The main regulator of bodily functions is a network of nerve cells known as the hypothalamus. This versatile organ is responsible for the basics of survival —guarding supplies of warmth, food and water, and managing reproduction.

To keep internal organs at their required temperature of 98.6° F., the hypothalamus has a thermostat monitoring the temperature of blood in the brain. When the body becomes overheated *(far right)*, the hypothalamus stimulates millions of sweat glands to produce perspiration, which emerges through the pores and evaporates to cool the skin.

Among its many other functions, the hypothalamus also serves as a triggering mechanism for release of crucial hormones by its appendage, the pituitary gland. These hormones govern growth, metabolism and sexual behavior. In women they control pregnancy by initiating the monthly ovulation cycle, and then stimulate the breasts to produce milk for feeding.

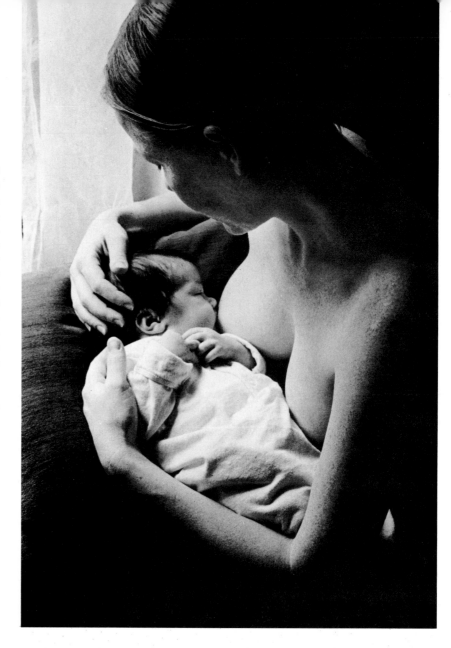

A mother nurses her baby with milk whose production was triggered by prolactin, a pituitary hormone released on signal from the hypothalamus.

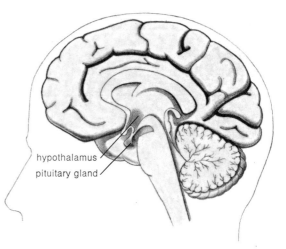

hypothalamus
pituitary gland

The bean-sized hypothalamus lies just to the left of the top of the brain stem. Hanging down from it by a half-inch stalk of nerve fibers is the pea-sized, hormone-secreting pituitary gland.

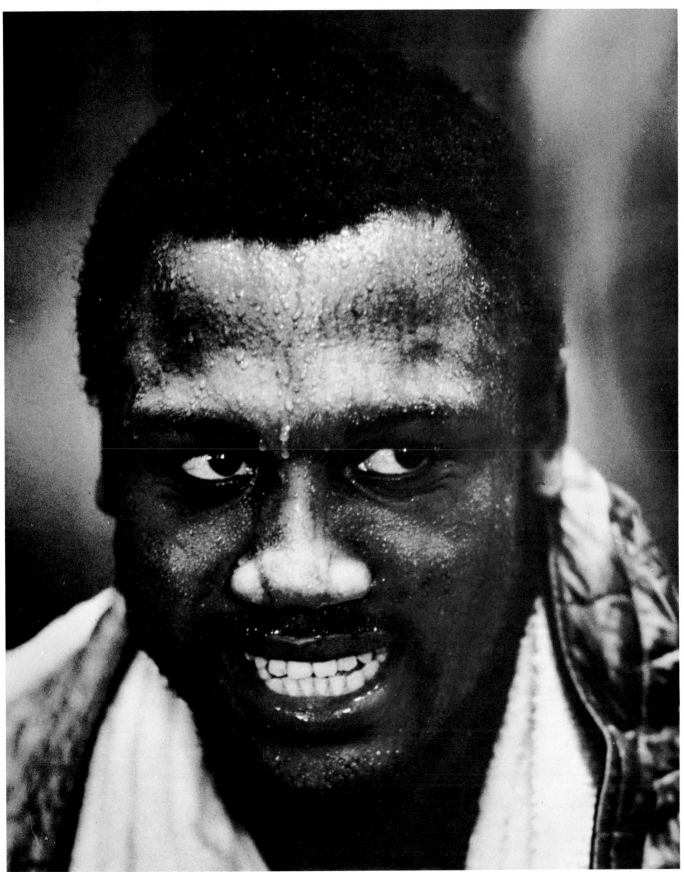

Perspiration activated by the hypothalamus cools the face of boxer Joe Frazier. If necessary, the body can sweat 12 quarts a day.

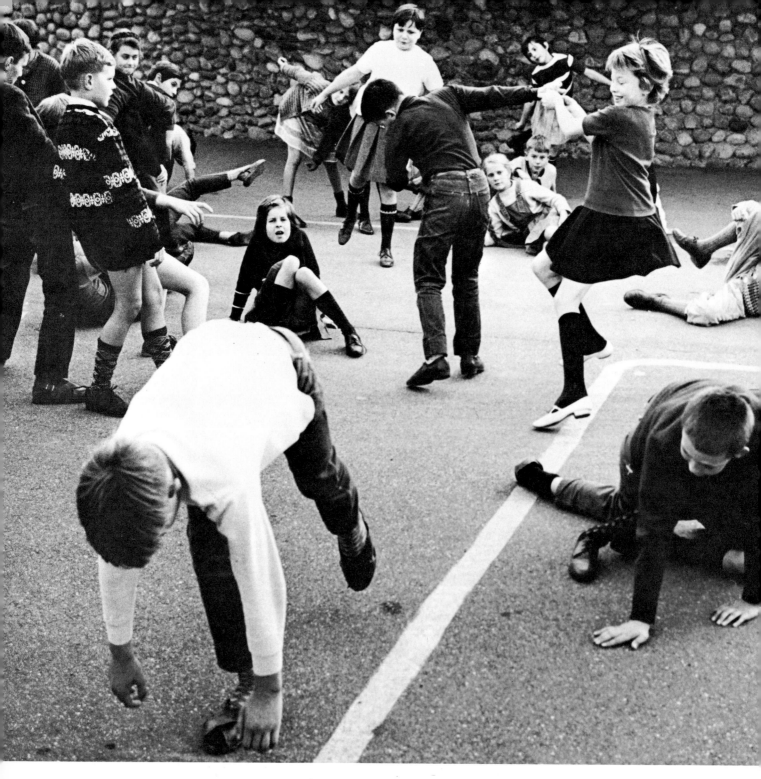

Making muscles act smoothly

The human body includes over 600 muscles, and every voluntary movement of them is initiated in the motor cortex, a band of nerve cells arching up over the top of the brain. Using electrical probes, scientists have mapped this area in detail *(page 19)*; their findings confirm the significance of two distinctive human traits: the largest areas control the hands, which give man his ability to use tools, and the lips, whose movements are essential to speech.

The motor cortex operates in conjunction with the sensory cortex *(pages 38-39)*, which provides necessary information about the positions and actions of various parts of the body. A key coordinator of these activities is the cerebellum, which refines body movements so that they work together.

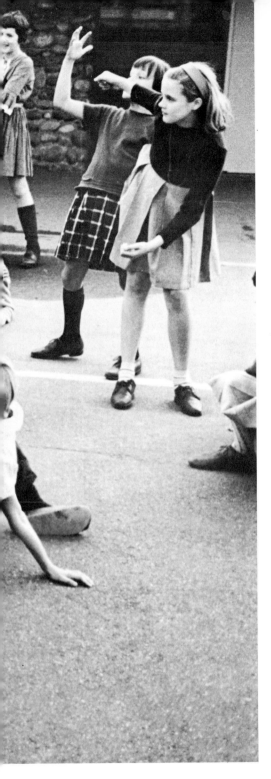

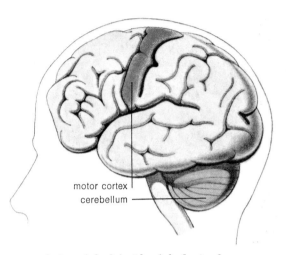

A view of the left side of the brain shows the motor cortex running across the top of the brain. Muscular activity is coordinated by the cerebellum, at the bottom of the brain.

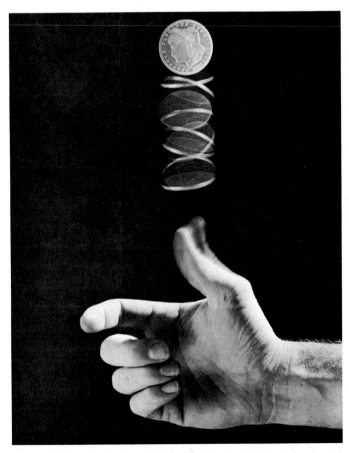

German youngsters put the motor coordination of cortex and cerebellum to the test, playing a game in which one child hurls another into a position he must hold like a statue.

Hand movements, like this flip of a coin, require such complex muscle activity that more of the motor cortex is devoted to one thumb than to an entire leg.

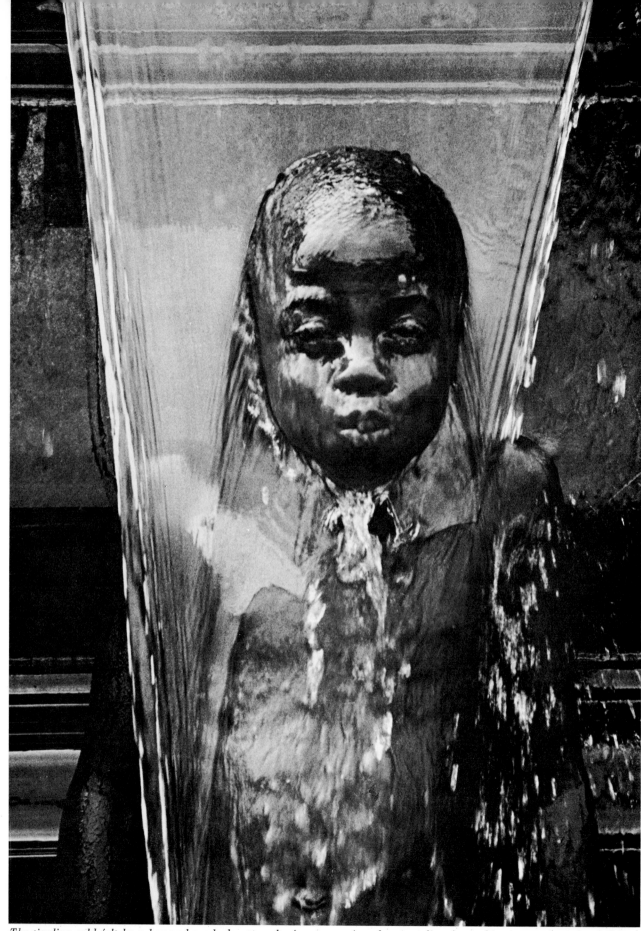

The tingling cold felt by a boy under a hydrant results from nerve impulses traveling from skin receptors to the thalamus.

A center of the senses

Everything that touches a human body, from the gentlest drop of rain to the sharpest winter breeze, sends nerve signals to the thalamus, traffic director for most sensations. It monitors and sorts signals, then sends them on to appropriate parts of the brain.

The thalamus relays eye impulses to the visual center and ear signals to the hearing center *(pages 40-41)*. A variety of body signals goes to the sensory cortex to inform it of positions and movement, enabling it, with the motor cortex *(pages 36-37)*, to regulate muscle action. But the chill of cold water *(left)* and the delicate finger pricks of Braille printing *(below)* apparently go to generalized thinking areas. Only one sense bypasses the thalamus entirely: Smell, perhaps the oldest and most primitive of all physiological perceptions, has direct connections to circuits in the centers of emotion in the limbic system *(Chapter 5)*.

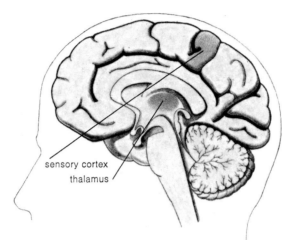

sensory cortex
thalamus

The thalamus, on top of the brain stem, collects, sorts and redistributes sense signals. Body sensations reach the sensory cortex, which helps guide muscles.

Forwarding information to his brain via tactile instead of visual impulses, a blind reader runs fingers over a manuscript in Braille, the internationally accepted system of writing for the sightless.

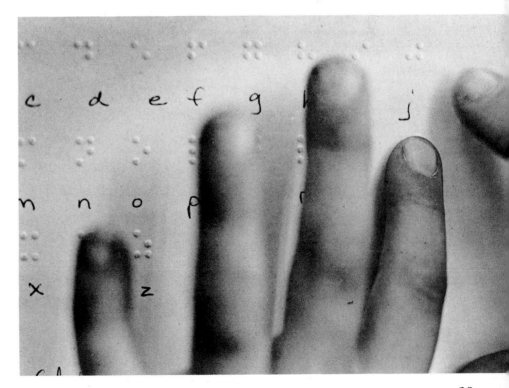

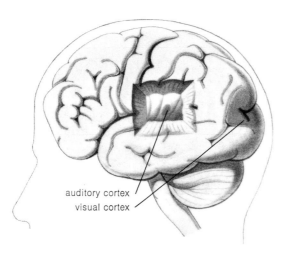

auditory cortex
visual cortex

A window in the brain reveals the auditory cortex, lying in the temporal lobe of each brain hemisphere. The visual cortex is in the occipital lobe, at the extreme rear of the hemispheres.

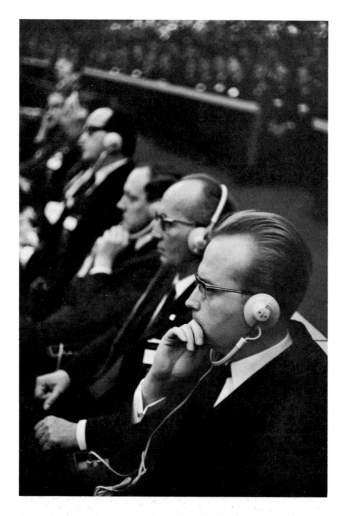

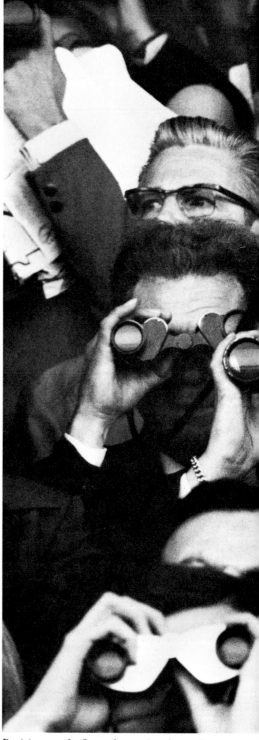

Parisians at the Longchamps track watch a race using human eyesight, nature's best all-around vision. Superior to a hawk's in every respect except distance-viewing, human sight is better at that too when aided by the binoculars in use here.

Businessmen at an international meeting in Germany listen to a simultaneous translation. If they also heard the untranslated original, the brain could conceivably understand both at once.

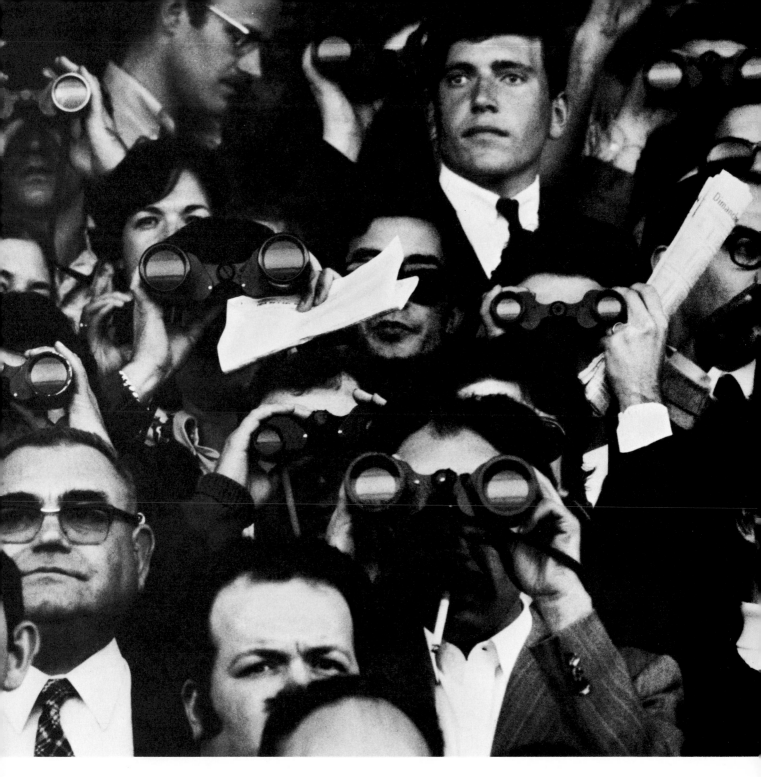

Interpreting sight and sound

Sight and hearing, the main senses that keep man informed of the world around him, are so important to human behavior that each has its own section of the brain as well as numerous interconnections to other circuits. Sight is generally the more delicate and reliable sense—a car may be heard approaching, but only visual perception reveals its course. And yet in odd ways hearing is superior.

The sound sense has one analytical capacity vision lacks. The visual cortex cannot distinguish among light waves—to see yellow and blue pigments in green, for example—nor can it readily pierce a reflected glare to perceive the view behind. The auditory cortex detects each instrument in an orchestra as well as their combined sound—and blocks noise outside to hear the music.

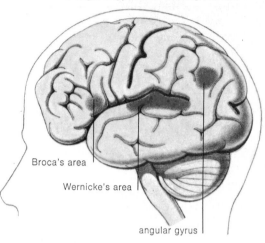

The brain's main speech centers are Broca's area, which controls the mechanics of speech, and Wernicke's area, which is the word retriever and selector. The angular gyrus is a linking station.

Broca's area

Wernicke's area

angular gyrus

Language centers of the mind

Man's distinctive skill is communication through language. Without this ability, he would be cut off from his fellow man, unable to learn or to profit from his experiences.

The crucial linguistic skill involves three connected centers in the brain. In Wernicke's area—named for the German neurologist Carl Wernicke, who discovered it in 1874—words are selected from the verbal memory. If the words are to be written, hand muscle controls go into action. If spoken language is required, signals are fired to Broca's area, named for *its* discoverer, Paul Broca of France; it stimulates regulators of the muscles in the face, lips, tongue and larynx.

The third center, the angular gyrus, is involved only when language depends on vision. It connects the visual cortex *(pages 40-41)* to Wernicke's area to call up words for things seen—and to permit the ultimate use of language in reading and writing *(right)*.

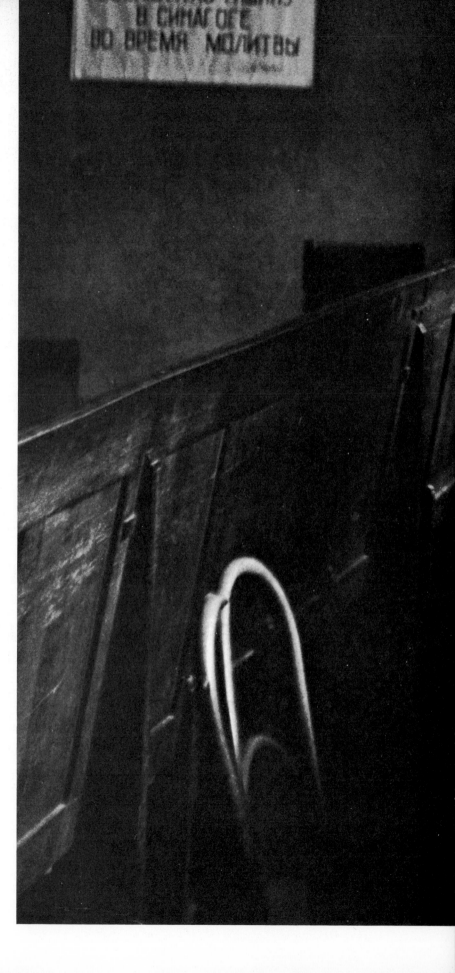

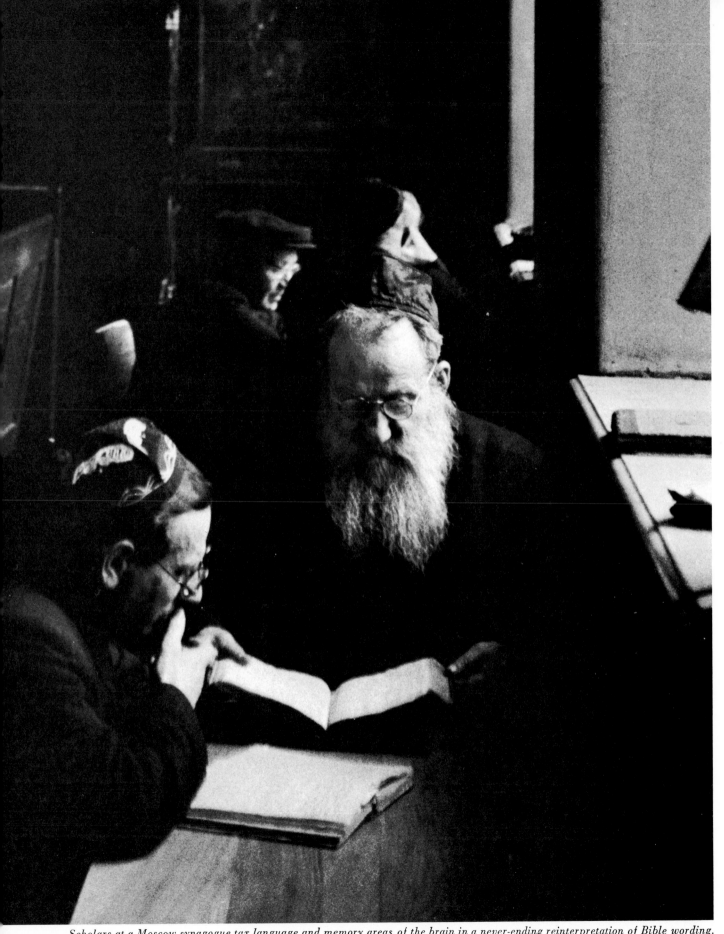

Scholars at a Moscow synagogue tax language and memory areas of the brain in a never-ending reinterpretation of Bible wording.

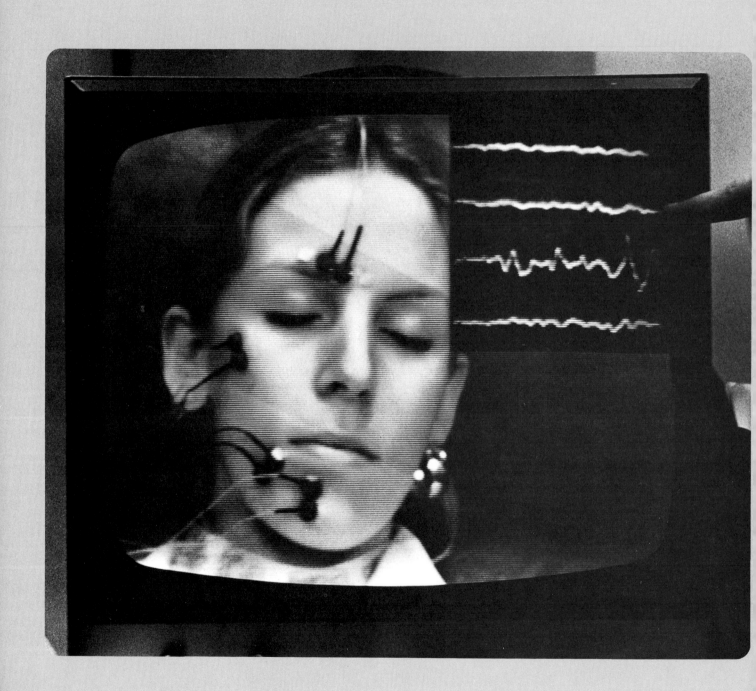

How the Wiring Works

2

The idea that the brain is a machine is hardly surprising. Understanding of its role grew with the expansion of science that accompanied the Industrial Revolution, and it was only natural to visualize brain operation in terms of man-made machines. In the 18th Century the comparison was to the clock, with its pulleys, cogs and gears. In the 19th Century, after the discovery that the brain uses electric signals, the comparison shifted to the newly invented telegraph and later, as technology advanced, the model became the telephone switchboard. One authority saw the brain as "an enchanted loom." More recently, the brain has been likened to the computer, the dazzlingly versatile calculating machine that can even be taught to play a game of chess.

In some respects these electromechanical models help explain the operation of the brain. Yet none of the comparisons is really apt. For the brain is far more intricate, more sensitive and more resourceful than any machine. It controls behavior with an immensely complicated electrical maze that contains millions of individual circuits. Each performs a function that may have been assigned to it by heredity or learned through experience—controlling movement in a set of muscles, sorting out the lines in the letter "Y," responding to a voice. These circuits, in turn, are made up of the brain's smallest working units, microscopic nerve cells, or neurons. Each person has at least an estimated 10 billion neurons in his brain. Most of them are so tiny that a cubic inch of brain matter contains up to 100 million neurons. Such small particles are the working units of the brain, the starting points for human behavior.

Neurons come in assorted shapes and sizes, resembling stars or misshapen balloons on a long tether, or uprooted trees with dense foliage on one end and an extensive root system on the other. The typical neuron has three essential parts: a cell body, which manufactures protein and other materials necessary for its own survival; a network of projections called dendrites (little fingers) that stick out a short way from one end of the cell body; and from the other side of the body one long, wiry axon, which branches out at its far end into a number of so-called terminal buttons. Under the microscope a stunningly beautiful view of the neuron is revealed when the specimen is treated with a solution of silver salts, using the Golgi method, which somehow stains only a few of the densely packed neurons in a slice of brain tissue. These few clearly defined neurons loom magically above their unstained neighbors, their tangles of dendrites and axons standing out in three-dimensional clarity *(page 49)*.

What the neuron does was fairly easy to figure out once Luigi Galvani announced the electrical nature of nerve signals—a discovery he made in the 1780s, when he connected his newly invented electric battery to the nerves of a dead frog and saw the frog's muscles twitch. Learning how those signals are generated and transmitted was more difficult, for the processes turn out to be fantastically delicate and subtle. Unraveling the mystery of why they operate the way they do is much more difficult but it is being accomplished. So far this understanding is speculative, but the speculations are now based on detailed information about the operation of neurons in controlling behavior.

The basic action of the neuron is called firing. The dendrites at the head of the cell body pick up a signal from a neighboring neuron, acting as a kind of receiving antenna. The signal changes the cell body's voltage—the strength of electrical force inside it. This voltage change travels along the axon, which functions as a transmission line, to the terminal buttons at the end of the axon. The terminal buttons act as a transmitting antenna, sending the impulse to another neuron.

By firing in this way the neurons control all operations of mind and body. When a man's finger encounters a piece of grit, touch-sensitive cells convert pressure into an electrical impulse. News of the encounter is quickly relayed to the brain by the successive firings of neurons; inside the brain, multitudes of other neurons fire in a flurry of electrical activity to weigh the significance of this news against other bulletins coming in from other sources—and against stored records of similar encounters in the past. If the new sensory information is judged worth pursuing, still other networks of neurons fire to operate muscles, which contract or expand when stimulated by electricity. These signals coordinate thousands of muscle fibers as the man turns his head, bends down and focuses his eyes on the small piece of grit that attracted his brain's interest.

The delicate mechanism that turns nerve cells on and off this way was analyzed by studying sea squids, which possess conveniently large nerves. So thick are some of the squid's axons—100 times the diameter of human axons—that when the English researcher J. Z. Young started working with them in the 1930s he mistook some for arteries. Later research by other scientists showed that each nerve cell is, in effect, a tiny living battery that periodically discharges and recharges itself.

Like all living cells, the neuron is completely encased in a microscopically thin membrane that serves as its skin. When the neuron is not firing, the fluid inside has a relatively high concentration of potassium atoms in their electrically charged form, potassium ions, and the fluid outside has a relatively high concentration of sodium ions. The cell has to work hard to keep these elements separate, because otherwise they would mix back and forth through the cell wall—as dissolved compounds separated by a membrane ordinarily do—until the concentrations on both sides of the wall were the same. How the cell accomplishes this feat is not known; apparently some agency in it controls the porosity of the cell wall. The process opens the pores that let sodium, but not potassium, ions out until the fluid concentrations are properly balanced; then the pores close. In effect, the cell pumps sodium out through a selective, adjustable sieve.

This pumping has an electrical effect because ions are electrically charged (potassium and sodium ions carry positive charges). The surplus of sodium ions outside the cell makes the liquid there positively charged. The deficiency of sodium inside the cell leaves that liquid negatively charged. But this state of affairs can change if the cell membrane is stimulated by an outside electrical effect—a minute increase in positive charge outside the cell. Then the membrane pores open again so that sodium ions can enter. The increased positive charge outside drives them back through the membrane, increasing the positive charge inside. The added positive charges do not counterbalance the negative charges there; they merely make the inside less negative than it was. This change, however, is enough to set off a nerve impulse. The cell discharges, releasing a burst of electricity. It then rebuilds the chemical and electrical differences to be ready to discharge again.

When this electrochemical change occurs in a neuron, it begins in a dendrite. A wave of electrical activity spreads out along the surface of the cell body like a ripple on the surface of a pond. When it reaches the axon, it gets caught up in a different reaction. The axon goes through a kind of flip-flop, reopening its pores first to sodium, and then to potassium, before returning to its original state. The electrical charge swings abruptly from negative to positive to negative again. Since the energy for this explosive reaction comes from the nerve cell itself, the neural impulse travels down the axon with undiminished vigor, much the way a flame travels down a fuse by constantly igniting the flammable material in the next section of cord. But while a fuse burns only once, the axonal membrane quickly recovers from the passage of an impulse, and after 1/1,000 second, it is ready for another.

The ability of the axon to transmit impulses fast is essential, of course, to get information rapidly to the brain and instructions back immediately to the muscles. In the human body nerve signals travel about 250 miles an hour. The speed depends partly on axon diameter; one reason the sea squid's axons are so big may be that the creature must transmit impulses at great speed to coordinate the system of jet propulsion that it uses to escape from predators.

If axon thickness were the sole factor in nerve speed, humans would be sluggish, slow-witted creatures or would require grotesque changes of anatomy to accommodate oversized axons. To get signals from eye to brain fast enough for clear vision under those conditions, the optic nerves would have to be 50 times their present thickness, and people would need much bigger heads. Fortunately, evolution provided a different solution. Thin axons can carry their electric messages rapidly because of a fatty white coating called myelin. It serves as insulation, like the rubber on electric wires, to prevent an axon from short-circuiting with the others that rub against it. This covering is very useful because the axon membrane is a poor insulator—about a million times leakier than the materials used on man-made cables. But the myelin does more. It has gaps, or nodes, at intervals, and these nodes speed transmission.

The myelin segments restrict the sodium-potassium changes to the nodes. At each node, the membrane is bared and the interchange of sodium and potassium can occur. It changes the electrical balance inside and outside the axon. And it is the electrical change in the liquid outside that is transmitted. It flashes along the outer surface of the myelin sheath to the next node, where it is regenerated to full strength and sent on again. Thus the electrical impulses of nerve signals do not travel inside the axon, like ordinary electricity in a wire, but zip along outside it. (The inside of an axon carries food supplies and is a very poor conductor of electricity.)

So critical is myelin to behavior that its absence markedly affects motor skills. The coating does not develop fully in humans until after the first year of life, delaying the appearance of such motor skills as crawling, and also bowel and bladder control—one reason early toilet training often fails. Myelin is vulnerable to the disease multiple sclerosis, which injures the soft coating. The damage to myelin throws

continued on page 53

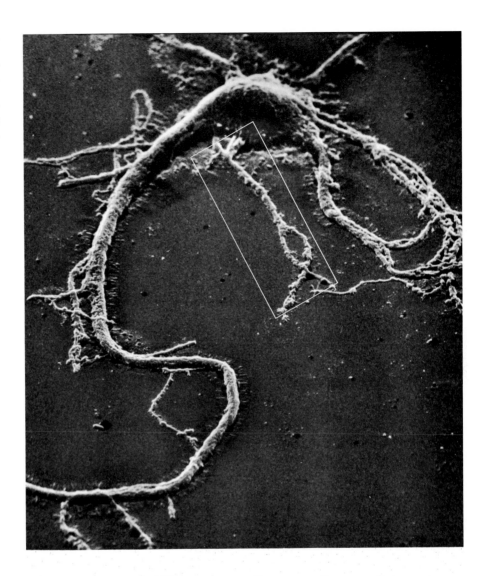

The muscle-moving circuits

The most basic step in behavior—the decision to move a muscle—begins in nerve cells like the one above. Its detailed portrait, made by Swedish photographer Lennart Nilsson with the aid of a complex instrument called a scanning electron microscope, is one of a series of extraordinary close-ups that show how the communications system starting in the brain controls every aspect of a human's existence.

Before a brain cell can order an arm muscle to move—perhaps to throw a ball—it and many like it must pick up the order from neighboring nerve cells. The message is a chemical change, de-tected by the twisting, branching fibers looping out of the bulbous cell body. The cell body weighs the order, count-ing the number and kinds of signals picked up. If the signals to fire predom-inate, the cell dispatches an electrical order down the axon *(white outline)* to release chemicals activating other nerve cells—which repeat the process, speeding the message on its way.

Through this quicksilver process, the message flashes down the main highway of the spinal cord to the place where the arm nerves intersect it, and mini-seconds later arrives at the appropriate arm muscle—to start the throw.

The routing system in action

From the brain's command center the message ordering an arm muscle to move flows into the spinal cord *(right)*, the main pathway to and from the brain. Packed into the pencil-slim cord are millions of nerve cells of many sizes interconnected along and across the cord *(right)*. They pass on messages —or stop them—according to the chemical influence of their neighbors.

Darting through this maze, the message to the arm muscle reaches a bundle of nerve fibers like the ones at left. These "peripheral" nerve bundles are similar to telephone cables, containing very long nerve cells with few interconnections. They make no decisions but simply relay the signal through their axons until each one branches off to a single muscle.

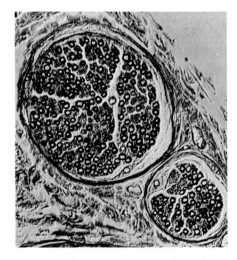

A cross section of two peripheral nerve bundles looks like a sliced telephone cable. The white dots are axons; the stained dark circles are myelin insulation. Each bundle is in a tissue sheath.

Pulled apart to show its complexity, a bundle of peripheral nerve fibers (above) relays messages between spinal cord and muscles. These nerves normally lie in long wirelike bundles with little branching.

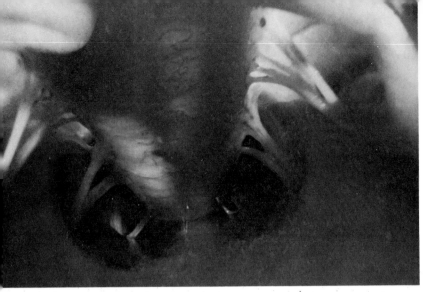

Looking down the spinal cord, this view
shows it entering the tunnel of the
vertebrae from the brain. At intervals
pairs of sensory and motor nerves feed
into it from various parts of the body.

A partial cross section of the spinal cord
at shoulder-blade height (below) shows
its intricate network of horizontal nerves
—bulky cell bodies, branching dendrites
and long axons—that supply extra
information for the vertical fibers
carrying messages to and from the brain.
This imput guides a moving arm and
times the release of a ball.

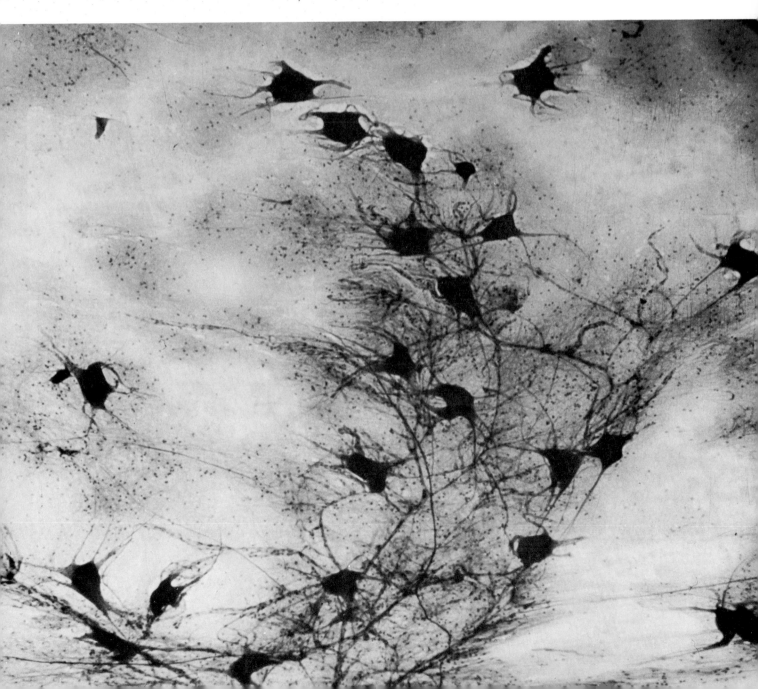

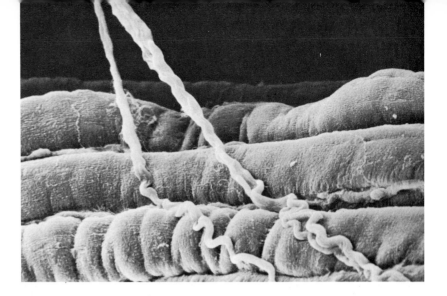

Magnified 500 times, three-twisted nerve fibers, each containing one nerve axon, cascade onto the undulating surface of a muscle and snake along its contours to deliver their action message.

The ultimate point of contact between brain and muscle is a flower-like cluster of sacs (below, right) at the end of a nerve fiber now stretched taut by its attachment to the muscle. From these sacs chemical stimulants flow to make the muscle contract—and throw the ball.

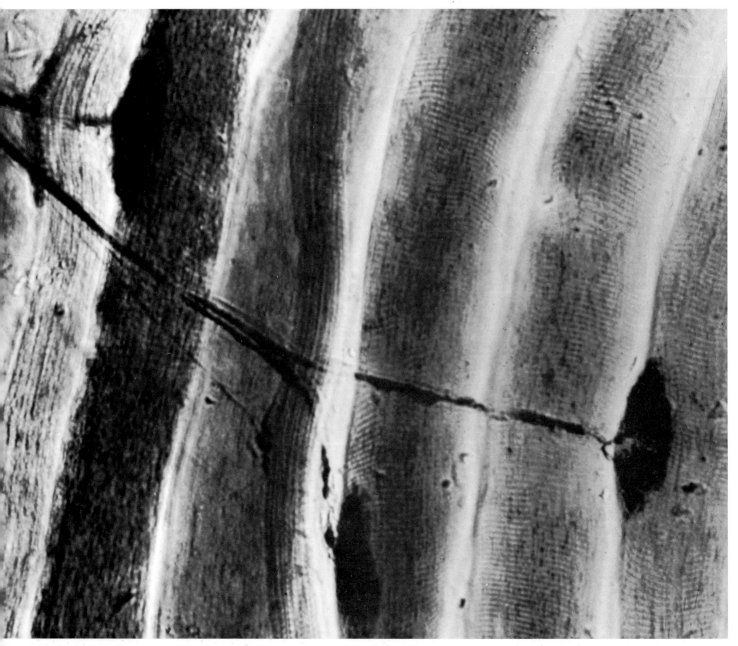

off the timing of nerve impulses and can cause jerky movements.

The production of myelin is one of the functions of a supportive group of brain cells called glia, which surround and protect neurons. Their name is derived from the Greek word for glue, for the glia cells seal up all the space around the neurons and seem literally to glue them together. In addition, the glia may screen out poisons from the blood that swirls around nerve cells but does not directly enter them.

This picture of a single neuron is relatively simple. A neuron becomes excited and chemically produces an electrical impulse that is generated again and again as it passes down the axon. The voltage of the impulse is always the same; only the frequency of firing changes. Even the rate of firing is limited—after each firing the nerve cell must rest for at least 1/20 second in order to recharge its chemical battery. It is hard to see how such an elementary scheme could account for the nuances of behavior. And if neurons worked only in this manner, man would be capable of nothing but the most mechanical actions.

The brain is not so simple, of course. It gets its power from an unusual feature of design. The brain's wiring does not run in a continuous web; neurons do not quite touch one another but are separated by unbelievably narrow gaps—eight millionths of an inch or 500 times thinner than the finest hair. These tiny clefts make possible the ingenious complexity and unpredictability of the human brain because they permit a great many permutations in connections between neurons. These connections, some permanent and some changeable, set up patterns to provide memory, control thought and regulate activity.

These breaks in the wiring, which occur where the tip of an axon almost meets the dendrite or cell body of another neuron, are known by a slightly inaccurate name—synapse, from the Greek word meaning clasp tightly. As recently as 70 years ago the very existence of the synaptic gap was fiercely debated. One group of scientists—led by the Italian Camillo Golgi, who invented the method of staining brain tissue for study under the microscope—said that neurons formed continuous electrical circuits. Golgi's leading opponent, the Spaniard Santiago Ramón y Cajal, took the Italian's staining method and used it to devastating effect —to infer the presence of the synaptic gap. Cajal's genius only heightened the rivalry with the equally gifted Golgi. In 1906 when the two scientists shared the Nobel Prize, they met on the rostrum to accept their awards but refused to speak to each other.

The discovery of the synapse may have settled one argument but it started another: how do electrical impulses manage to cross the gap? On one side were the "spark" theorists, who said the nerve impulse simply leaped across the synapse, much as electricity jumps the gap in an automobile spark plug. Opposing them were the "soup" champions, who maintained the impulse was not strong enough to jump a synapse; it had to be carried across by some chemical.

The first good evidence that this chemical action was the correct explanation emerged in the early 1920s from the basement laboratory of an Austrian chemist named Otto Loewi. The idea for the crucial experiment came to Loewi one night in a dream. He woke up, scribbled down his inspiration and went back to sleep. The next morning he could not decipher his own handwriting. That night he had the same dream, woke up while the insight was still clear in his mind and rushed down to his basement to begin the experiment. Loewi worked with frogs. He knew that certain nerve fibers that terminated in the heart always retarded the frog's heartbeat when they fired. So he stimulated these fibers in one frog, immediately collected the fluid from the heart of the frog and transferred it to the heart of another frog. The second frog's heart slowed down, just as if Loewi had stimulated its nerves. Evidently those nerves secreted a substance, later identified as acetylcholine, that influenced the firing of other nerves.

Today scientists know that acetylcholine is only one of 11 such chemicals that they believe serve to bridge the synaptic gap. Each neuron contains tiny sacs of one of these neurotransmitters just inside the tip of its axon. Release of the chemical is triggered by the electrical impulse traveling down the axon. A very tiny amount of the chemical—a few thousand molecules—shoots out of the cell, crosses the synapse and bombards the membrane wall of the other neuron. If the transmitter is an "excitatory" type, it alters the permeability of the membrane so that sodium can enter the cell, setting off the crucial exchange of sodium and potassium and creating an electrical impulse. If the transmitter is, like acetylcholine, an "inhibitor," it changes the pores of the membrane to keep sodium out and prevent firing.

Neurotransmitters have a dramatic influence on behavior. The poison curare, used by South American Indians, blocks the action of certain neurotransmitters and prevents the passage of nerve signals, causing paralysis and then death by suffocation. Other drugs—notably marijuana, LSD and amphetamines—also create their effects by tampering with the transmitter chemicals. And many serious ailments also seem to be caused by either too much or too little of a particular transmitter. Parkinsonism, a disease that causes a progressive loss of muscular control, apparently results from a lack of a transmitter called dopamine. Severe mental illnesses have been related to an imbalance of the transmitter serotonin. High blood pressure is sometimes connected to an overabundance of still another transmitter, norepinephrine. All of these ailments have been successfully treated with drugs that restore a normal supply of the transmitter involved.

Discovery of the action at nerve connections—transmitter chemicals making signals leap the spaces at synapses—helps explain the intricate flexibility of brain operation. Some neurons have axons that branch out to form synapses on thousands of other cells. And a single neuron may have as many as 200,000 synapses. In one cell several different transmitter chemicals may be bringing signals in across thousands of synaptic connections. The possibilities are enormous. One combination of signals from eyes, ears, memory and thinking circuits may trigger a cell in the network for tears; a slightly different combination would not. The cell, bombarded at thousands of synapses by conflicting orders, some saying fire, others saying do not fire, must decide. It takes a vote. Somehow it counts the yeas and nays during a given time period and responds accordingly. A simple majority of yeas will not make the cell fire its electrical impulse. The majority must be large enough to boost the cell's voltage to its firing threshold—like firewood that must get very hot before it bursts into flame. When the cell fires, it is in turn casting its own vote at synapses with other cells. One authority estimates that the cells in the brain make 500 trillion synapses—enough yes and no votes, it appears, to account for the endless permutations of human behavior.

By making synaptic connections, neurons form circuits, or pathways, that carry out precisely defined functions. Even the simplest of these circuits, involving only a few neurons, intersect in vast grids that can be imagined only by multiplying a millionfold the intricacy of a spider's web. A human's instantaneous act such as stepping back from an oncoming car brings into play numerous grids of interconnecting pathways involving as many as 100,000 neurons—circuits for seeing, hearing, feeling, memory and movement. In some portions of the brain and nervous system circuits can be mapped virtually neuron by neuron.

The easiest circuits to trace are, of course, the motor circuits, because it is so easy to see if a stimulus is having an effect. And the easiest motor circuits to work with are those that control certain motor reflexes—automatic movements that do not originate in the brain.

The simplest stretch-reflex circuit, for example, consists of only two nerve cells—a sensory neuron and a motor neuron—connected by one synapse. The best known stretch reflex is probably the knee jerk, which doctors often test to see if there is some defect in the nervous system. Doctors use a little rubber hammer to tap the knee just below the kneecap, but anyone can try the test on himself by crossing his legs, relaxing them and tapping below the kneecap of the raised leg with the edge of his hand. The leg jerks up instantly, as if by its own will. The response is so powerful that in one unfortunate experiment, in which the reflex was stimulated electrically, the subject suffered a broken leg.

The knee-jerk circuit forms a simple loop. Tapping the knee stretches the muscle and triggers an impulse in a sensory nerve wrapped like a tentacle around part of the muscle. The impulse races up the nerve axon, through the nerve cell body and out along another section that extends into the spinal cord. There it makes a synapse with a motor neuron. The synapse excites the motor neuron, setting off an impulse that shoots down that axon to tell the muscle to contract and jerk the leg up. The impulse from a single loop of this kind cannot do the job. Probably hundreds are involved, but all of them are simple two-neuron, one-synapse pathways. The stretch reflex has other, more complex tasks. It enables muscles to adjust to sudden changes in load without orders from the brain. When a cowboy in a TV Western leaps onto the back of his horse, the horse's stretch reflex keeps the animal from collapsing under the sudden load.

Reflexes are generally automatic. The brain can get involved, however, and control them if absolutely necessary. The hot-stove reflex, for example, ordinarily guarantees instant withdrawal of a finger from a burning sensation. When a nerve in the finger screams "Hot!" the electrical message courses through that nerve's long axon up the arm, through the cell body and into the spinal cord. It reaches the spinal cord at a point just below the motor neuron that can deal with the problem. So the signaling nerve makes a synapse with an intermediary neuron, which in turn connects with the motor neuron and orders the finger to pull away. This response is generally automatic. Fast action is obviously necessary to prevent serious injury, and the signals take a shortcut instead of going up to the brain and down again. But the brain can override this reflex.

Intersecting with the circuits of the hot-stove reflex, which can automatically remove the finger, are circuits from the brain that provide conscious, voluntary control of finger movement. Thus the wiring exists for the will to countermand the reflex's automatic order.

An extreme situation in which the brain might overrule the hot-stove reflex is provided by the British scientist Steven Rose in his book *The Conscious Brain.* "Suppose someone is holding a revolver at one's head —move the finger and he shoots," Rose suggests. At such a moment, he

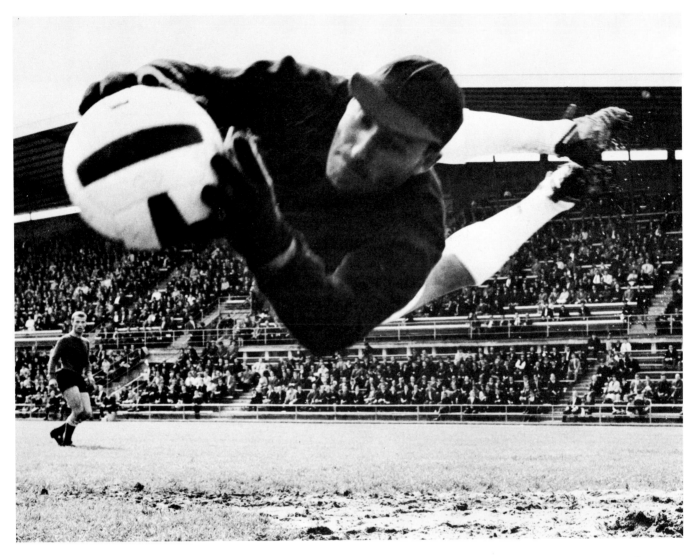

Swiss goalie Hans Stedtler leaps to trap a soccer ball. After years of practice, Stedtler performs the complex action almost without conscious thought; according to one theory, his brain's cerebellum directs the whole sequence of activities involved in leaping and grasping, sending a single command from the supervisory motor cortex.

explains, the brain nerve cells intervene. " 'No, leave it there,' they say, 'or worse will befall.' " The reflex circuit's neurons would tend to excite the motor neuron; the brain circuit's neurons would inhibit its firing. Presumably, the nays would have it.

Automatic reflexes account for only a few of the body's nerve circuits. Most muscle movements are voluntary; the individual consciously controls them through tracts of nerve pathways that extend from the brain through all regions of the body. The main tract descends directly from the wrinkled layer of gray matter at the very top of the brain, known as the motor cortex.

The motor cortex contains more than a million unusually large nerve cell bodies, most of them pyramid-shaped. Descending from them, a million axons snake down the spinal cord, making connections with neurons that in turn control individual muscles in the trunk and limbs. If the spinal cord is severed by injury or disease, neural impulses between the brain and any part of the cord below the break are interrupted. Paralysis and loss of feeling result, though reflexes controlled from below the break, such as the knee jerk, soon resume functioning.

Scientists have mapped the circuitry of the motor cortex with astonishing precision. The map shows just which patch of cortex controls which muscular activity. The amount of cortex devoted to various parts of the body clearly demonstrates the two main traits that distinguish man from his fellow animals. By far the largest areas of motor cortex are allotted to just two features of human anatomy: the hands, reflecting the vast number of neurons necessary to coordinate intricate manual jobs such as writing with a pencil; and the mouth, including the tongue, jaws and throat, all of which are necessary for the coordination of man's highest faculty—speech.

Right next to the motor strip is the sensory cortex, its nearness suggesting the importance of sensation in the voluntary control of movement. Anyone whose foot has fallen asleep knows how hard it is to make precise movements without being able to feel muscles moving.

The motor cortex does not control muscle movements all by itself. New techniques for probing beneath the surface of the brain have revealed that other command centers work in tandem with the motor cortex. In one experiment indicating the importance of these secondary centers, a monkey was first taught to flex the right wrist and hold it flexed for one second while, through a very fine microelectrode, scientists recorded the firing of single cells in the monkey's brain. Just before the monkey flexed its wrist, a neuron in the motor cortex fired. But so did neurons in at least two other parts of the brain—the basal ganglia and the cerebellum. Both areas are connected, either directly or through roundabout circuits, to each other and to the motor cortex. By observing the effects of damage in each area, scientists have been able to ascertain the role each plays in coordinating muscular activity.

The basal ganglia apparently play a fundamental role in initiating movements, like reaching down to pick up a burden. It is this area of the brain that is now known to be affected by Parkinsonism. The nerve cells of the basal ganglia fire too rapidly, resulting in a bizarre combination of muscle tremors and rigidity. The misfiring is caused by an insufficiency of an inhibitory neurotransmitter called dopamine; and a drug, L-Dopa, dramatically relieves the disease, apparently because it is taken up by neurons in the basal ganglia and converted into the dopamine that the brain needs.

Coordinating movements, like touching the tip of your nose, seem to be the province of the cerebellum. For a long time the cerebellum was relegated by researchers to an ill-defined back-seat role in the control of muscular activity. But they have now learned that it is wired not only to the motor cortex and the basal ganglia but also to an impressive array of sensory apparatus—the eyes, the ears, and especially the long nerves that alert the brain to every movement a muscle makes. When a person reaches out to shake hands with a friend, the cerebellum somehow computes the relative positions of the two hands and automatically guides the hand and adjusts its speed for a smooth greeting. If the cerebellum is damaged, the friendly hand reaches out but begins swinging about wildly, unable to zero in on its target. Damage to the cerebellum also affects the ability to walk, and victims of cerebellar disorders lurch so erratically that a few have been arrested because the police thought that they were drunk.

Electrical stimulation of the cerebellum sometimes relieves muscular ailments that may originate elsewhere in the brain. One example is dystonia, a hereditary disease in which opposing muscles tense at the same time, locking an arm or hand in a painful position. One New York brain surgeon, Irving Cooper, has helped dystonia victims by implanting on the cerebellum tiny electrodes, which are powered, like a heart pacemaker, by a battery pack worn on the belt. The trickle of electricity to their cerebellums helps keep their muscles from locking.

Of all the behavioral command centers, the cerebellum is the only one with circuits so straightforward in their connections that scientists have traced in them what an electronics engineer would recognize as a wiring diagram. The neurons are arranged in precise patterns that repeat themselves over and over again, like printed circuits in a computer. Of course, just being able to draw a wiring diagram does not necessarily explain why the cerebellum works the way it does, any more than tracing the paths of all the colored wires in a telephone switchboard explains how the telephone system works. Nevertheless, a British scientist, David Marr, has used the wiring diagram as the foundation for an ingenious theory about cerebellar function; he argues that the cerebellum is a recording machine that tapes muscular actions involved in complex and habitually used movement and then plays back entire sequences on command.

In trying out new skills for the first time, a person tends to think through and consciously order each movement—a process that presumably takes place in the higher brain centers. These consciously thought-out commands are fed through the cerebellum; its circuits perceive the

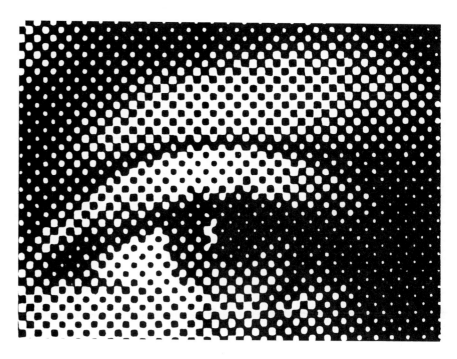

The brain helps the senses by filling in gaps, supplying information the sense organ may not record. The eye does not see a smooth image but registers a scene as a pattern of dark and light spots, like those visible in the enlarged photoengraving above. The brain somehow melds the dot pattern into continuous tones.

higher cerebral activity and instantaneously reproduce it, like a ballet student who mimics the steps his teacher is demonstrating. In time, the cerebellar circuits no longer have to watch; they take over the precise coordination of the skilled movements, so that the individual need not bother to think about the details anymore. Thereafter, nerve cells in the motor cortex can simply switch on the cerebellum's playback mechanism and get the same result—much as pushing the button on a tape recorder plays back a song. Marr says the cerebellum is able to learn such kinetic melodies because the synaptic connections between repeatedly fired neurons become stronger and more effective with practice. The more often a particular nerve circuit is used, the fewer the mental operations needed to set it up for use again.

Scientists hope that new techniques of electrical and chemical stimulation will enable them someday to trace all the diverse circuits involved in movement. This research might lead them to those cells that signal a person's intention—his will—to make a particular movement. Many experts believe these cells are located in front of the motor cortex, in the lobes in the front and sides of the head. Injuries to these lobes can turn intended movements into charades of meaningless repetition. The Russian psychologist A. R. Luria cites such cases among patients who suffered war wounds: the man who kept on trying to strike a match after it was already lit; another who planed completely through a piece of wood and went on helplessly planing through the workbench.

A do-it-yourself experiment demonstrates the role of these intention

Sometimes the brain's attempts to help the senses backfire and produce misinformation. In the pattern above, the gray spots barely visible at the intersections of white lines are an illusion, arising from the brain's effort to perceive shapes by heightening contrasts. Where white is bordered by black it appears whitest. But where lines of exaggerated white intersect, the tiny blocks where they meet seem gray by comparison.

centers on movement. Close one eye and tap a finger very gently on the corner of the other; the room will appear to jiggle because the eye movement was not ordered directly by the brain—no intention to move was signaled to the vision center. In ordinary eye movement, the muscles of the eyes are willed to move, and the room does not jiggle. Voluntary eye movement apparently involves *two* sets of signals, both originating in the mysterious centers of intention. One signal tells the eyes to move. The second tells that part of the brain concerned with seeing to disregard any signals that show the room jiggling. In most movements the complex interrelationships of many brain centers are necessary to achieve the remarkable feats of muscle coordination that people usually take for granted. No matter how a person signs his name—fingers cramped at the bottom of a personal check or hand and arm scrawling letters in chalk two feet high on a blackboard—the signature always bears his unique, unmistakable stamp.

The wiring of muscle-control circuits, labyrinthine though it may be, relies on comparatively simple types of nerve cells and synaptic connections. The brain's sensing apparatus is much more complex, perhaps because, while motor action is usually directed at a single object, perception must keep the individual informed about a great number of things at once. So far as brain mechanisms are concerned, sight is the most important sense. What a man sees—or rather what he thinks he sees—represents up to 90 per cent of the brain's input of sensory information at any one time.

Each eye is constantly transmitting news over a million separate channels. Light enters and is projected onto light-sensitive cells, some 130 million of them. Most are slender rod shapes that respond with hazy images and only to black and white but are so sensitive they work in starlight. A small group in the center, cone-shaped, are the only ones that distinguish colors and fine detail—but they are too insensitive to work even in moonlight. Inhibition plays a big role in the action of these cells. They maintain a steady background firing rate even when the eye is in total darkness. When a spot of light falls on a small patch, certain cells are excited into a rapid rate of firing. But other cells are inhibited and decrease their firing rate. These groups of "on" and "off" cells are so arranged that their responses exaggerate the difference between a brightly illuminated area and a dark area. This scheme guarantees that the individual will be aware of the contours that define shapes against relatively featureless backgrounds—such as the contours that help distinguish an obstacle in the dark.

This information from the rods and cones is interpreted only in the vi-

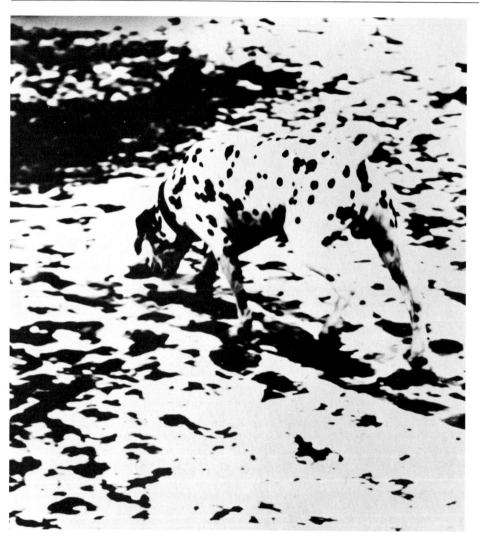

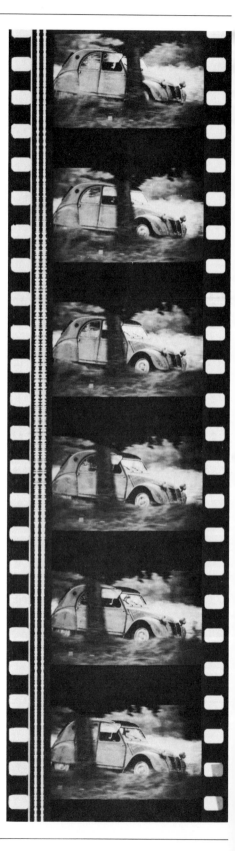

Useful flaws of the brain

The brain's ability to fill in gaps—and sometimes to fool itself in the process—has practical consequences. One is camouflage, a method of concealment that is based on the brain's tendency to gloss over distinctions between closely related patterns and to assume the larger pattern continues. This camouflage effect causes the brain to lose the dog above against its spotted background.

A modern application of this trick of the brain is the movies. Eye and brain fill in the gaps between the frames so that stationary pictures seem to move.

A dalmation blends into a dappled background because the brain first registers the overall pattern of the animal and its surroundings rather than the dog's outline. Either concentration or movement by the animal reveals the difference.

When these still pictures are flashed on a screen at 24 frames a second, with intervals of darkness between frames, the viewer sees a moving car. The illusion arises because the eye continues to register each image after it goes off, missing the intervals between. The brain blends the figures into one moving image.

sual cortex, the mind's eye. Just as the firing pattern of on and off cells in the eye emphasizes one feature of the visual field, neurons at higher levels are arranged to pick out more and more complex features from the firing patterns of lower-level cells. For example, a brain neuron may be wired so that it fires only when a certain number of on cells, arranged in a straight line in one corner of the eye, are simultaneously activated. This kind of brain neuron is a line detector.

The existence of such pattern detectors was suspected from the experience of victims of severe migraine headaches. They often perceive intense visual displays at the beginning of an attack. Apparently nerve cells in the visual cortex start firing spontaneously, producing in the victim's vision spectacular arrays of bright bars and corners of light —called fortification illusions because they resemble an aerial view of old-fashioned military fortifications. More than a century ago a British physician concluded from his own migraine displays that they represented a realistic record of electrical fireworks in his brain. His intuition has now been confirmed by numerous experiments.

The specific jobs of many neurons in the visual cortex have been painstakingly sorted out in animal tests by two scientists at Harvard, David Hubel and Torsten Wiesel. They insert a microelectrode into a single cell in the visual cortex of a cat or monkey. Then they flash patterns of light and dark onto a projection screen in front of the animal. They have found cells that increase their firing rate only in response to a line displayed at a precise angle in a particular part of the field of vision. Other cells respond to any line as long as it is tilted at the proper angle. Still others respond to more complex patterns such as corners and curves. Certain cells fire rapidly only if the line of light moves across the projection screen. (A similar motion analyzer is found in the frog's eye, where it acts as a bug detector to aid the frog in catching its main food, flying insects.)

It is not difficult to imagine how pattern detectors enable people to read. Line-detector cells might work together to sort out simple shapes such as the letters of the alphabet. The letter Y, for example, consists of three lines, each at a particular angle. A set of line detectors, each oriented differently, could pick it up. But in order for the brain to recognize this shape as a Y, there would have to be another set of neurons that responds only when the line detectors are simultaneously stimulated by a vertical line that branches off with two slanting ones. And what happens when a person finds the letter Y followed by the letters E and S, and immediately recognizes the combination as a word? Does this mean that there is not only a group of special neurons for detecting each letter in

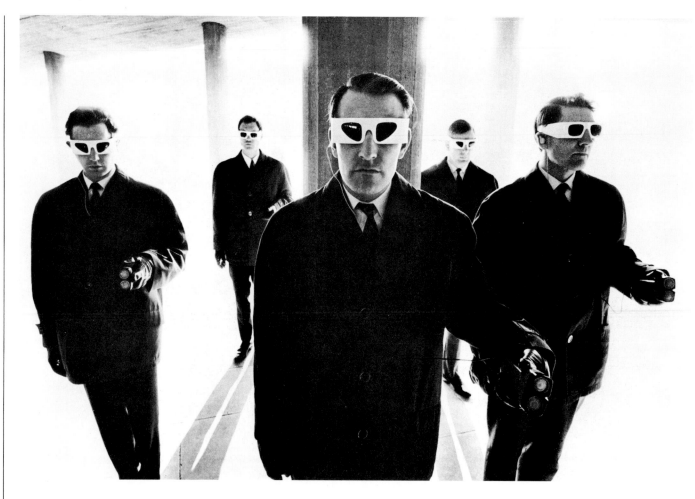

Wearing opaque glasses to block vision, British researchers test a device that might someday enable blind people to use hearing circuits in the brain to guide walking. The "sonic torch" in each man's hand bounces high-pitched sound waves from solid objects and makes a beep in an attached ear piece to warn of obstacles.

the alphabet, but also special neurons for immediately recognizable words like "yes," "no," "and," "of"?

Logically, it would seem that the chain of pattern detectors must end somewhere. But at the moment scientists have no way of knowing how far back the chain can be traced. One researcher has found a neuron in a rhesus monkey's brain that responds only when the monkey is shown a silhouette of the hand of a rhesus monkey. A silhouette of the hand of any other kind of monkey provokes no such response.

Conceivably, a rhesus monkey might be born with a cell prewired for the job of recognizing the hands of other rhesus monkeys. But if there are pattern-detecting neurons for shapes like the letter Y, it is clear that such cells must learn to respond in this manner. And this would imply that the brain has some way of storing a model of the letter Y in a set of neurons, so that future perceptions can be compared with the model until something triggers an "Aha!" neuron—a cell that fires only when a newly perceived pattern closely matches a previously stored pattern.

Evidence that the brain regularly stores complex visual patterns for instantaneous recall comes from an easily observable phenomenon of the visual pathway—the so-called blind spot of the retina. The blind spot occurs at the point where the axons from the eye's light-sensitive cells gather in the back of the eye to form the optic nerve that carries signals to the brain. At this spot no light-sensitive cells are found. Anyone can locate his own blind spot by closing one eye, staring at the wall and moving a pencil slowly across the field of vision. At the blind spot the pencil tip briefly disappears. People are ordinarily not aware of this hole in the field of vision because some mechanism in the brain automatically fills in the gap. It calls on its store of patterns to provide part of a pattern that the eye missed. The only people who can literally see this pattern-recalling mechanism in action are those who suffer from the large blind spots called scotomas, which sometimes appear during migraine headaches. The memory researcher Karl Lashley liked to tell stories about his own migraine attacks. One migraine blind spot was so big that it momentarily beheaded a colleague who happened to be standing in front of Lashley. Without an instant of doubt, Lashley's brain obligingly filled in the gap—but it plucked the wrong pattern from the store and supplied, instead of a man's head, vertical stripes from the room's wallpaper.

Presumably, pattern detectors, infinitely more complex than those that recognize lines, control the elaborations of human behavior. Somewhere in the brain there must be a circuit of nerves that fires when the ear picks up the notes of a Bach concerto. Somewhere else there must be another circuit that fires only when the first fires, turning off other similar circuits that identify the notes of Beethoven or Brahms. And somewhere else there must be still other detector circuits that fire only when the recognized notes are enjoyable.

A few of these more complex brain responses can be traced—pleasure centers have been located in the brains of a number of animals, for instance. But no one has yet analyzed the wiring that enables a man to think and create—to sit down at a desk and pencil musical notes that will not only make his own brain say "Good!" but elicit the same thought in the minds of other people. The whole brain may be involved. But once the creative impulse has germinated, a familiar process is set in motion. The command sections of the brain—motor centers or whatever, depending on the kind of action involved—send out signals, and the basic brain mechanism is triggered. Neurons begin to fire, spreading impulses through the body to fingers, ears, eyes, arms, legs—and thought is translated into action.

When the circuits misfire

One of the most poignant and trying afflictions that can affect the lives of children and their parents is cerebral palsy. The result of the destruction of cells in the brain, it strikes about 15,000 infants a year in the United States alone. Because brain cells do not regenerate, the damage is irreparable, and the various disabilities that can be brought on by cerebral palsy—among them impaired speech, sight or hearing as well as floppy, spasmodic movements and mental retardation—are lifelong.

The damage can occur before birth if disease or infection harms the fetus, through a mishap during birth, or through accident later. In the case of the six-week premature baby at right, Esme Farb, the trigger was a condition called hyperbilirubinemia, a build-up of excess bile pigment. The ailment can be dangerous for any baby, but is especially so for a premature infant whose liver may not be sufficiently developed to filter out the bile pigment. If high concentrations of the pigment get into the bloodstream and are carried up into the brain—as happened with Esme—they can damage or kill vital cells.

The region apparently most affected by Esme's attack of hyperbilirubinemia was the basal ganglia, which is located deep in the middle of the brain and which contains motor control centers. As a result, Esme's body movement is uncoordinated. She also cannot talk coherently and she has other physical defects *(next page)*. But her parents, Nathan and Judith Farb, did not despair. And as Nathan's pictures on the following pages show, wise care and training have done much to offset the brain-damaged child's incapacities.

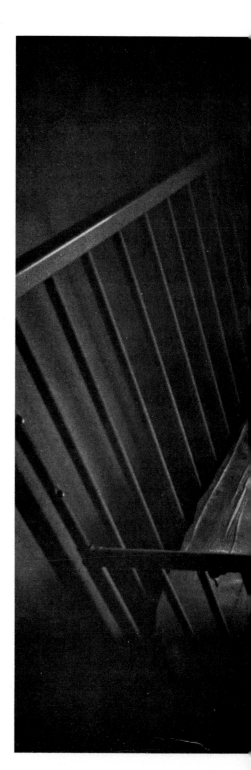

In her first hour out of an incubator, Esme Farb lies quietly in a crib in a Montana hospital—18 days after she was born prematurely while her parents were on a camping trip. At this time the Farbs already knew that she probably had defective hearing, discovered when she responded irregularly to a bell-ringing test. And a neurologist had warned them possibly to expect other disabilities that can accompany cerebral palsy.

PHOTOGRAPHED BY NATHAN FARB

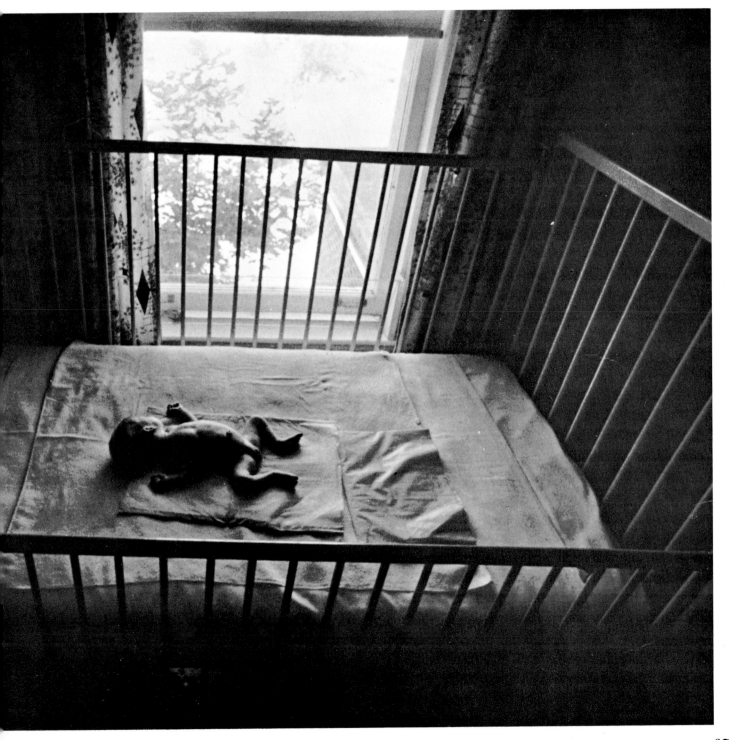

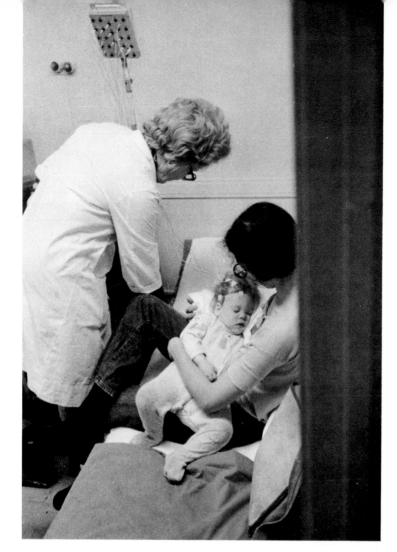

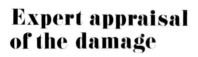

Being tested for epilepsy at 16 months, Esme dozes in her mother's arms while a technician readies an electroencephalograph, a device that records electrical activity in the brain. The test showed no trace of epilepsy.

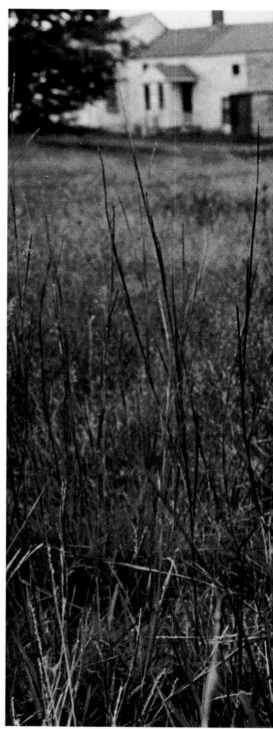

Expert appraisal of the damage

After the Farbs came home to New York City, they began a round of neurologists' offices while keeping a close watch on Esme's development. The physicians observed the slow spasmodic muscle responses—known as athetosis —that indicate the type of cerebral palsy originating in the basal ganglia.

Esme also suffered a diversity of other symptoms, suggesting that brain damage extended beyond the basal ganglia. She had difficulty balancing her body, was somewhat deaf and could not focus her eyes properly *(right)*. And she was slower than most premature babies in developing motor skills; even at seven months she could not sit unsupported for more than a minute or two before she helplessly toppled over.

*At one year, Esme strains to coordinate
her eye movements, trying to focus on her
father's camera as he takes her
photograph following a large reunion the
family held in Underhill, Vermont.*

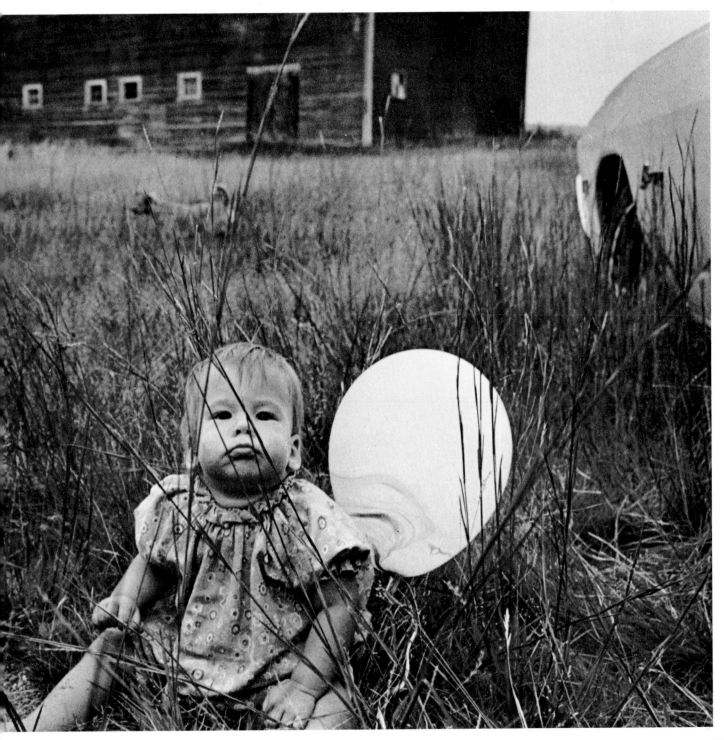

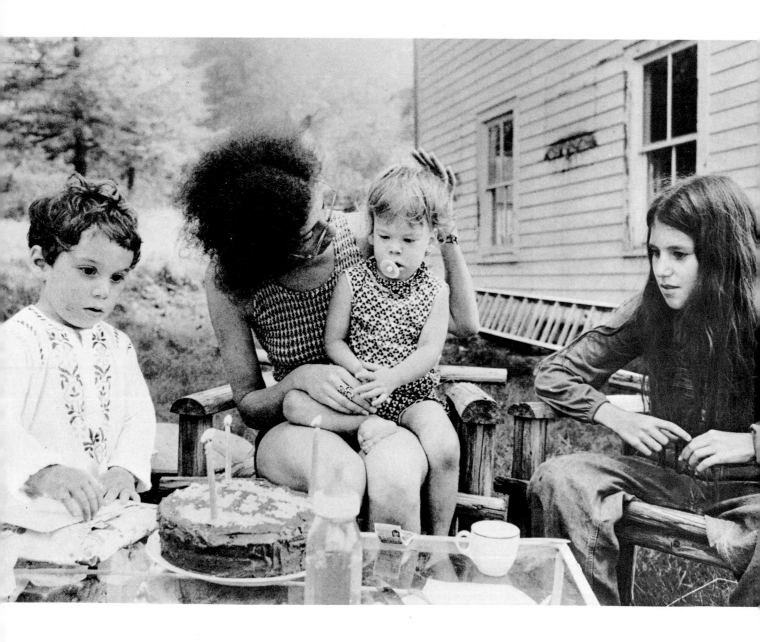

"Pushing us apart, pulling us together"

By the time she was two, Esme could solve visual puzzles that did not depend on any knowledge of language. This achievement reaffirmed the Farbs' belief that her IQ was normal, an evaluation that her doctors later supported. But she could neither walk nor talk, abilities most children begin to develop around the age of one.

The Farbs' concern over Esme, plus the strain of taking care of her, brought on a painful period of discouragement. In weathering it, they learned that Esme was the center of family life. Says Nathan, "Sometimes she pushes us apart, but usually she pulls us together."

Puzzled by her birthday cake, Esme sits on her mother's lap, between a playmate (left) and her older sister Ruth, and stares uncomprehendingly at its candles —two for her years and one to grow on.

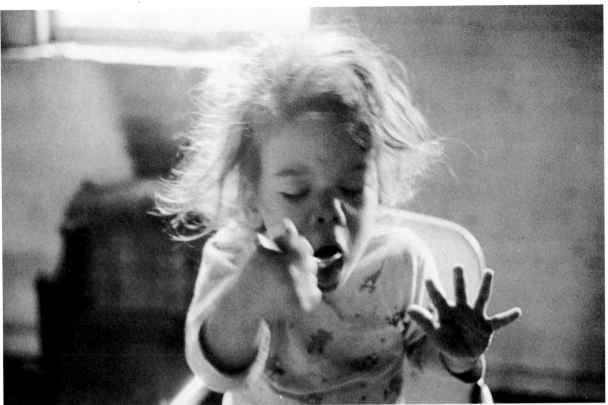

Esme raises both arms to keep from spilling food out of a spoon. Using a fork was easier because she could spear food.

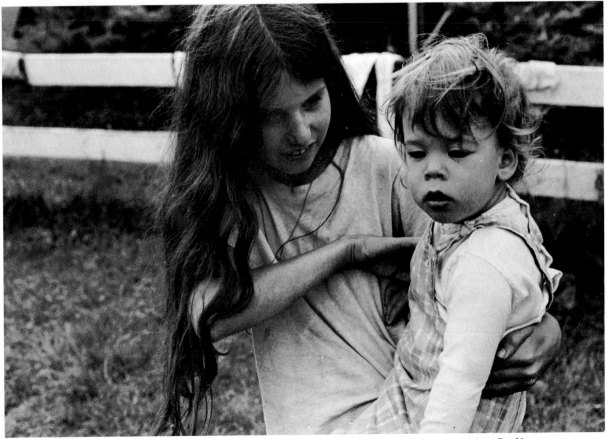

After repeated requests brought no response, Esme is turned to the camera by Ruth during a visit to Ruth's summer camp.

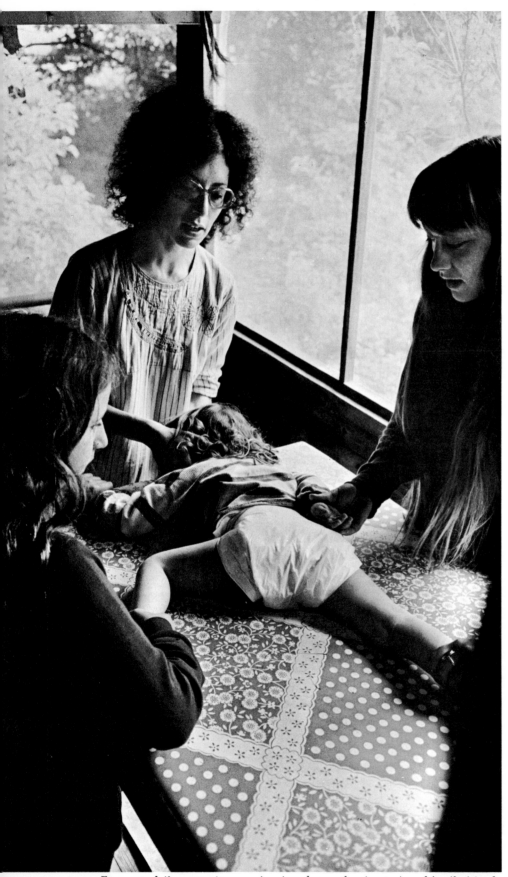

Grasping at therapeutic straws

As Esme grew older, the Farbs tried a variety of approaches to improve her condition. To counter her deafness, they had her fitted with a hearing aid. They followed routines that they hoped would develop the potential of her undamaged brain cells; to stimulate body sensations, for example, they bathed her in alternating hot and cold water, then rubbed her with a rough towel.

But one major problem remained: Esme's inability to walk. To strengthen her muscle coordination, Judith Farb gave her swimming exercises. To improve her balance, the family taught her to somersault. They also used an exercise known as patterning *(left)*, in which the child's head, arms and legs are moved in a crawling motion. The exercise is supposed to plant a pattern in the brain so that the child will start to crawl properly—and later walk unaided. Most rehabilitation authorities say the method is useless and even the Farbs are divided on its value. Mrs. Farb thinks it helped her child, but her husband wonders if Esme would not have made the progress she did *(following pages)* without it.

Esme gets daily patterning exercises from her mother (center), and family friends.

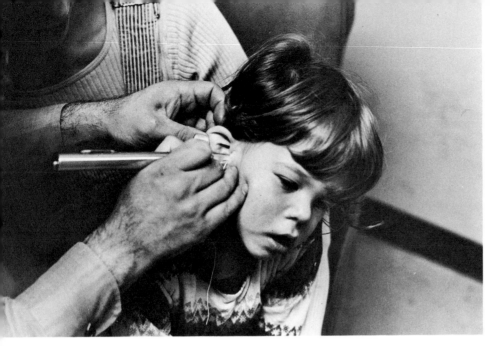

A technician to whom the Farbs were sent by the New York League for the Hard of Hearing takes a wax impression of the inside of Esme's ear, the first step in making her a hearing aid.

At a weekly, three-hour parent-child guidance class, Esme eats with her classmate, with whom she was paired because both functioned at similar levels. The youngsters are observed by their mothers (right) and two staff members.

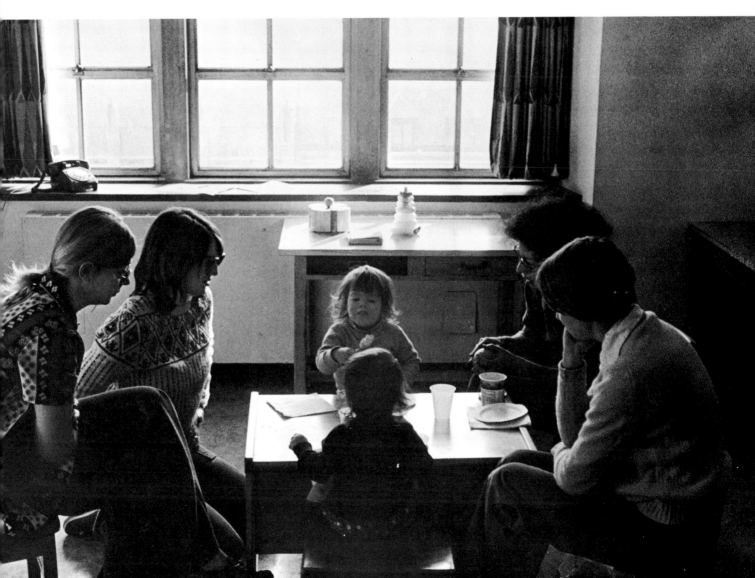

Tentative steps toward a better life

It was not until Esme was 30 months old that she finally began to walk unaided. Along with this physical progress, she displayed a growing personality—she was playful, attentive and persistent. She was also enterprising: Since she was unable to say more than a few words, she taught her family a sign language she had worked out, patiently using each sign until they caught on to what she meant. For example, if she wanted her hearing aid, which she wore hung on her chest, she pointed to her chest with one hand and her ear with the other. To indicate "Where is it?" she flung her arms out wide.

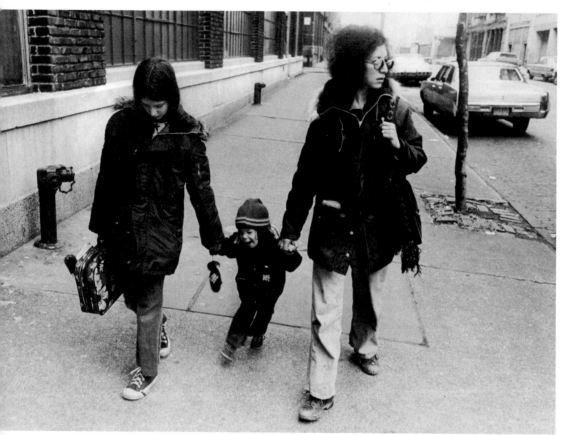

A few weeks after learning to walk, Esme takes a stroll down a Manhattan street with Ruth and Mrs. Farb. At this stage she still has an occasional tendency to slip into a somewhat knock-kneed gait.

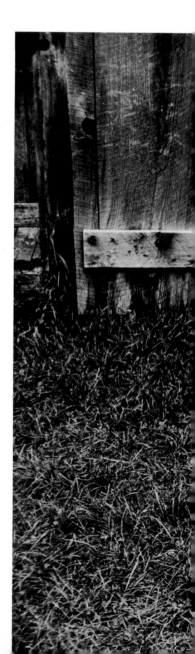

Sturdy and merry at three years old, Esme chortles with glee (right) as she attempts to hold a badminton racquet that is several sizes too large for her during a game in the country with one of her sister's friends.

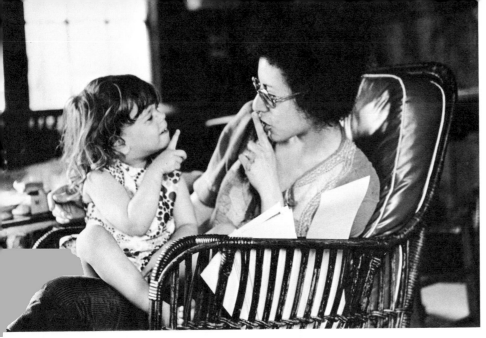

Teaching the sign she uses to mean someone is asleep, Esme watches (left) as her mother puts a finger to her lips. But therapists have urged the Farbs to discourage Esme's use of signs and to insist that she learn to talk.

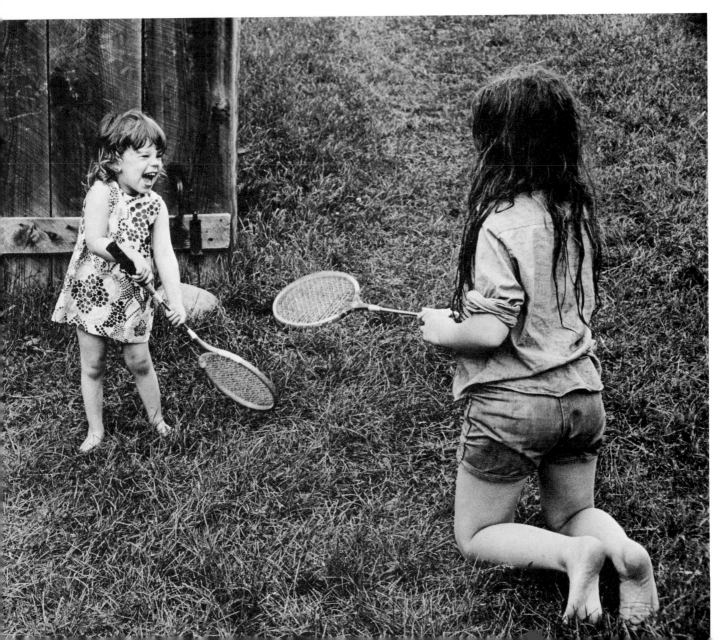

Coming out into the world

The Farbs were determined above all that Esme, though physically handicapped, should grow into an emotionally healthy, outgoing person. Accordingly, they decided to expose her to social experience outside the family circle by enrolling her in a nursery school for normal children when she was three. She was put in a class with two-year-olds, spending three days a week with them and the other days at home doing speech and movement therapy.

When Esme's classmates had trouble understanding the way she talked, they accepted the fact calmly. As for Esme, she proved to be decidedly gregarious, making friends easily and readily adjusting to school procedures. In two months she was advanced to a class with children her own age. To the Farbs, it was a hopeful sign that Esme will be able to adjust successfully to the world that exists around her.

Momentarily alone and disoriented (below), Esme watches the other children clamber up a slide in the schoolyard. When she first tried the slide herself, she slid on her back, but in a few weeks she learned to slide the way everyone did.

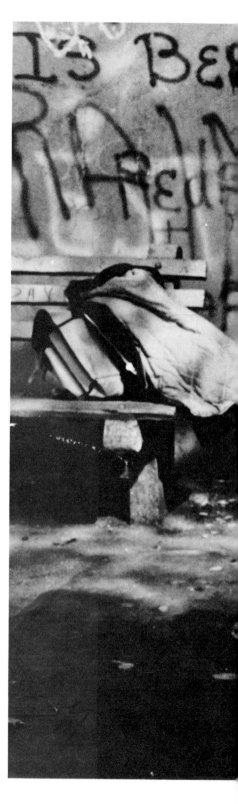

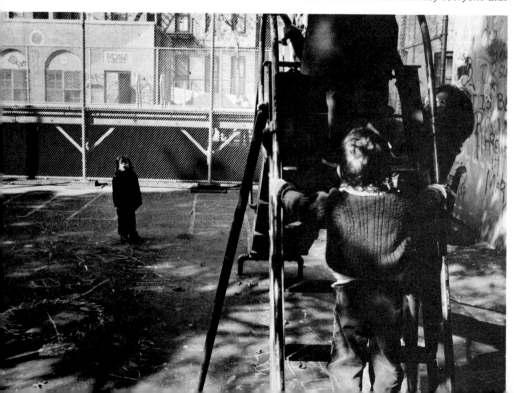

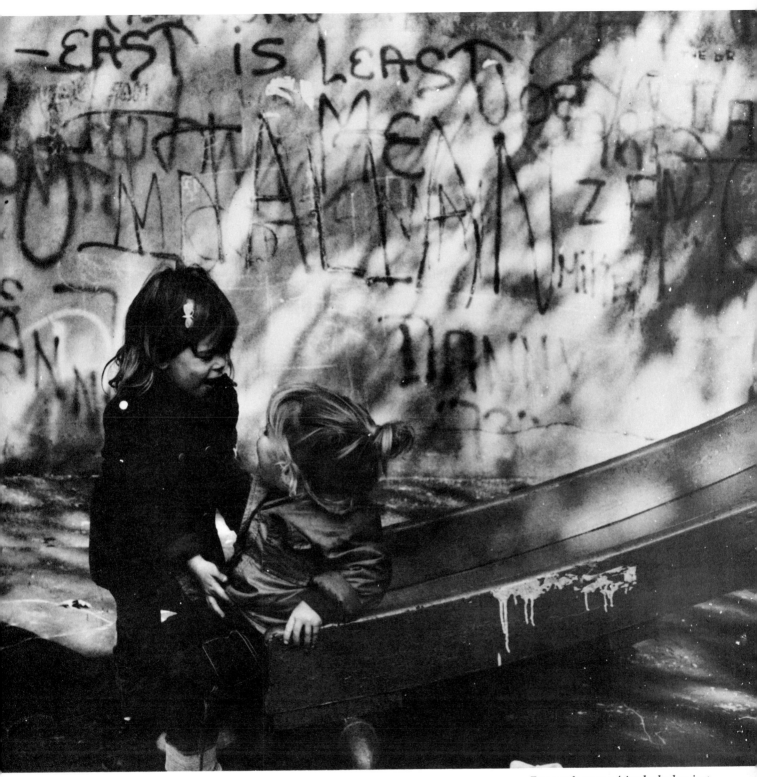

Esme welcomes a friend who has just come shooting down the slide, expressing her good spirits in nonverbal but understandable physical actions.

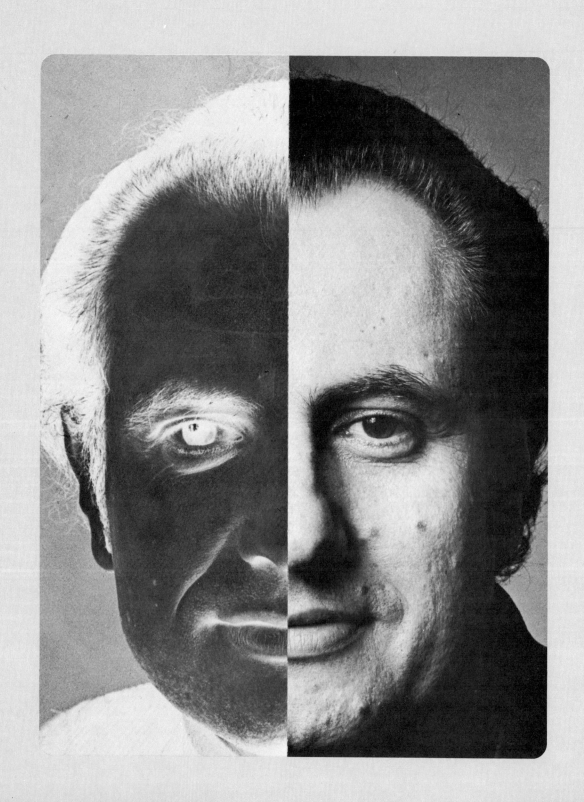

The Split Brain

Everyone has two minds. Most people feel that way occasionally, but only recently have scientists learned how accurately this subjective impression mirrors physical reality. There are two brains. Perched atop the brain stem inside the human skull are two large bulges—the left and right cerebral hemispheres. Ordinarily the two are interconnected so that they work together, sharing the work of the brain, and each can, if necessity demands, take over many of the functions of the mind as a whole. Yet the two brains are not alike, and a number of crucial responsibilities are divided between them. They have quite different roles in behavior. The left brain, highly literate and analytical, tends to dominate personality. It specializes in language skills such as speech and writing, as well as in mathematics and reasoning. The right brain, endowed with special powers of intuition and spatial perception, is particularly important to creativity, music, art and athletics.

The location of intellectual talents in the left brain was deduced over several centuries of autopsy examinations that revealed damage to the left side of the brain in people who, through illness or head injury, had lost the ability to speak or calculate. But only recently have the specialties of the right brain—and many crucial distinctions between the right and left brains—come to light. This knowledge arises mainly from studies of patients who, for medical purposes, have undergone operations to sever the main connections between their two brains, the corpus callosum. This bundle of nerve fibers, 1/4 inch thick and 3 1/2 inches long, permits information received in one hemisphere to be perceived by the other also. When it is cut, the autonomy of the two brains becomes dramatically apparent. The impact on behavior in certain experiments is astonishing, though ordinary behavior is hardly affected. Each on its own can think, learn and remember. And each is capable of feeling such strong emotions that the two minds sometimes struggle for supremacy as if they were distinctly different selves.

The division of responsibilities is unique to the human brain. All vertebrates also have twin hemispheres in their brains, but the hemispheres are truly twins, each capable of doing whatever the other does. An animal that damages one side of its brain loses some general capacity without losing any particular mental skill. Not so a man. Since his hemispheres are, in many crucial respects, specialists, damage to one —by the blood clots of stroke, for example—may eradicate an essential group of capabilities. In some cases the lost capacities can be relearned by the unharmed hemisphere, but only laboriously.

The most familiar example of a cerebral specialty is handedness. About 92 per cent of all people use only their right hands for the most delicate physical tasks, such as writing, and favor the right when strength is required. Their left hands and arms are clumsier and weaker. Because the nerve circuits that connect most muscles to the brain cross over before they enter the brain, the left hemisphere controls movements of the right side of the body. Consequently, right-handed people use their left brains for most physical work whereas most left-handed people use their right brains.

The favoring of one hand over the other makes good sense, though it is not clear why the right should be favored so predominantly. Evolution emphasized manual dexterity, and the ability to hold an object in one hand while working on it with the other was clearly a great advantage to early men. They were able to use this ability more efficiently because of the division of labor between the brain's two hemispheres. The development of the precision control that goes with the favoring of one hand can be seen taking place as a child progresses; not until he is around one year old does he learn to hold a toy with one hand and manipulate it with the other hand.

Even more specialized is the brain's management of man's unique gift, language. The ability to write and speak almost always resides in one hemisphere; in 97 per cent of the world's population it is the left hemisphere—even most people who use their left hands and right brains to control the physical movements of writing use their left brains to determine what they write.

Since language represents the brain's highest function and is the most distinctive feature of human behavior, its localization in the left brain caused scientists until recently to focus their research on that hemisphere and to label it the major hemisphere. The nonspeaking right brain, meanwhile, was relegated to a back-seat role, and called the mute, or minor, hemisphere. How wrong this downgrading was is only now being realized.

Evidence that the right brain possessed special—and valuable—pow-

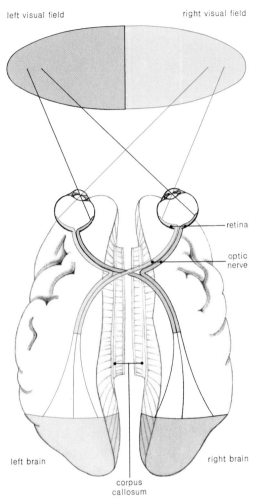

How a split-brain patient perceives different images in each brain is indicated above. Cells in each eye are normally divided so that one group looks to the right, the other to the left. The nerves cross so that the left view of both eyes goes to the right brain, the right view to the left. If the patient keeps his eyes still, each brain gets but one view—and his cut corpus callosum prevents an interchange. In laboratory experiments performed on cats—whose eyes cannot be kept still—some optic nerves must be cut.

ers had long existed, but few scientists had paid much attention to it. One clue appeared as early as 1745, when a physician described a patient whose left-brain language center was badly damaged by a stroke. He could not "say a single word except 'yes' and has to communicate by making signs with his hands." But strangely, the writer noted, "He can sing certain hymns, which he had learned before he became ill, as clearly and distinctly as any healthy person." This observation, it is now known, is one indication that singing and other musical abilities are a right brain function.

In 1864 another neurologist suggested a second power of the right brain—certain capacities of visual perception. The Englishman Hughlings Jackson observed that a woman with a tumor in her right hemisphere had lost this capacity. He reported, "She did not know objects, persons and places."

These extraordinary findings went largely unheeded and untested for nearly a century. The accepted wisdom was that man had one brain, ruled by the talkative left hemisphere. But then came a decade of experiments that rank among the most remarkable in the history of brain research. Known as the split-brain studies, the work began at the University of Chicago and later shifted to the California Institute of Technology. These investigations demonstrated that the right brain, far from being a minor hemisphere, influences significant aspects of behavior. Moreover, they showed with bizarre clarity that each person does indeed have two minds.

In the beginning, such possibilities scarcely occurred to the chief researcher, Roger W. Sperry. He had already made a name for himself by demonstrating the precision with which heredity wires the nerve circuits of the brain. Now, he determined to investigate visual perception and the mechanism by which visual information is transmitted and stored in the brain.

Sperry suggested to one of his graduate students, Ronald Myers, that he study visual learning in cats, and Myers set out to find how the cats' two eyes and two brains influenced their ability to acquire new skills. Normally, in cats as in humans, a large area is seen by both eyes, but within each eye, the right side of the retina picks up from the left and the left side from the right. Each side of the retina in each eye has its own group of nerve fibers leading to the brain, and they divide before they get there. The nerves from the right side of both retinas—the sections looking to the left—end up in the right brain; the nerves from the left side of both retinas go to the left brain. Thus each half of the brain receives a different image—the right brain sees the left part of the view and the left brain sees the right part. Ordinarily the two images are combined mentally, with the help of the corpus callosum interconnection, to give what appears to be a single view in depth. Myers decided to change this scheme surgically, so that each of a cat's two brains would receive signals from only one eye rather than from both.

What Myers did was to cut into the optic nerves, leaving intact for the left eye only the bundle of fibers that linked it to the left brain. Similarly, he cut into the other optic nerve so that the right eye's impulses were carried only to the right brain. The effect was that each brain had its own eye—left brain left eye, and right brain right eye. Myers then cut the corpus callosum, the bundle of nerve fibers that normally interconnects the two hemispheres *(diagram, page 81)*.

At this point, Myers was ready to test how this splitting of a cat's vision and of its brain affected its behavior. By offering and withholding rewards of food, he taught the split-brain cat to discriminate between a circle and a square with its left eye only—the right eye was covered. Then the left eye was covered and the cat's right eye was shown the circle and square. A normal animal that had learned the problem with one eye would have been able to discriminate between the forms with the other eye, since visual signals would have reached both hemispheres of the brain, and they were also interconnected by the corpus callosum. But the split-brain cat showed no sign of recognition. It was as though the cat had never been exposed to the problem. The animal had to be taught all over again to discriminate between the two forms with the right eye. The cat, in effect, had two brains, functioning independently of each other.

In other experiments split-brain cats were taught to make opposite choices with each eye—a square with one, a circle with the other. When the right eye was blindfolded, the left eye learned that a square meant food and a circle meant no food. When the blindfold was shifted to the left eye, the right eye learned to identify the circle with food and the square with no food. The cats learned to follow these conflicting instructions without the slightest evidence of confusion, further proof that their disconnected left and right hemispheres were operating as independent and entirely separate brains.

The discovery that a split-brain cat could use either of its two brains independently prompted Roger Sperry and his colleague, Michael Gazzaniga, to investigate the behavior of humans whose brains had been similarly split. Such operations were not new at this point. As early as the 1930s neurosurgeons had been trying to relieve the effects of severe epilepsy with a variety of brain treatments. They had cut chunks out of var-

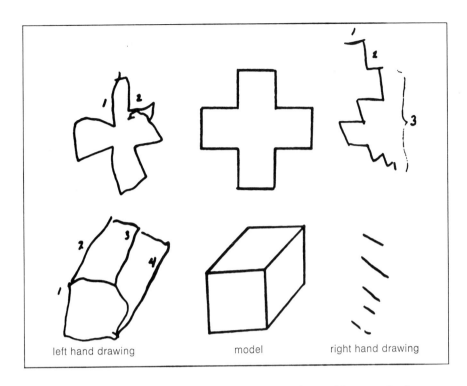

left hand drawing   model   right hand drawing

ious parts of the brain in attempts to limit the wild spread of nerve signals that sets off a seizure. Then they hit upon the idea of cutting the corpus callosum, the major carrier of nerve impulses between the brain's left and right hemispheres. The callosum's importance was not known at this point (one neurophysiologist suggested jokingly that its sole purpose was "to keep the hemispheres from sagging"). But the surgeons thought that if the callosum were cut to separate the hemispheres, seizures might be confined to one hemisphere and thereby limited. The operations proved remarkably successful, virtually eliminating the attacks. Apparently the callosum had served to intensify the effect of the seizures by conveying the aberrant nerve signals from one hemisphere to the other.

Although disconnecting the callosum almost totally eliminated the worst seizures, it produced no noticeable changes in temperament, personality or general intelligence. One patient, a 12-year-old boy, awoke brightly from the operation and, though complaining of a "splitting headache," was quickly able to repeat the tongue twister "Peter Piper picked a peck of pickled peppers." Another patient, a 48-year-old veteran of World War II whose seizures had started when bomb fragments penetrated his brain, said he felt better than he had in years. He was interviewed by Roger Sperry, who commented, "In casual conversation over a cup of coffee and a cigarette, one would hardly suspect that there was anything at all unusual about him."

While humans with split brains seemed normal, Sperry and Gazzaniga knew that split-brain cats could act in extraordinary ways. They decided to probe more deeply into the behavior of the human patients and devised special tests to restrict the information reaching one side or other of the subject's newly bisected brain. In the case of information gained through the sense of touch, this routing was simple. The objects that were used in the test were kept hidden behind a partition so that the subject could not see them. He would grasp an object such as a spoon or comb with one hand. The only information reaching his brain came from this hand's sense of touch, and it reached only one of the two hemispheres, since touch nerves from one side of the body are connected to just one hemisphere—right hand to left brain, left hand to right brain. There could be no communication between the two hemispheres of the brain because their interconnection had been cut. Thus, if the patient felt the object with his right hand, his left brain would know about it but his right brain would not.

Visual tests presented more of a problem. In the experiments on the split-brain cats, it was possible to cut parts of optic nerves *(diagram page 81)* so that images seen by one eye were transmitted to only one hemisphere. For the tests on humans, the researchers obviously could not tinker with the optic nerves. Instead, they simply asked the patient to look straight ahead without moving his eyes and flashed a very brief image to one side, so that it could be seen only by one side in each retina and would therefore register only in one side of the brain. A picture flashed off to the left would be picked up only by the right sides of the retinas in each eye and would register only in the right brain.

The tests quickly showed the subtle dichotomy of the split brain—and confirmed beyond all question the specialization of the left brain in language skills. In one test the subject was required to fix his eyes straight ahead on the midpoint of a board while lights were quickly flashed left and right. Lights that flashed into the right half of his visual field, and thus were seen by his left brain, were easily reported by the subject—because his left brain is the hemisphere controlling speech. But when lights were flashed into the left visual field it was as if the subject were half blind. The right brain saw the lights but, lacking speech, remained mute. However, when the patient was asked to point to where the lights had been, he had no trouble indicating their position: the right brain can control physical movement.

In another experiment, a printed instruction telling one of the split-brain subjects to move his left hand was flashed into his left visual field. There was no response. His right brain received the message but could

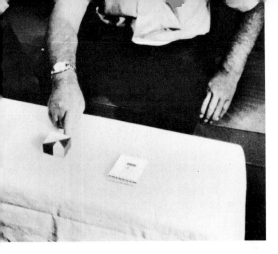

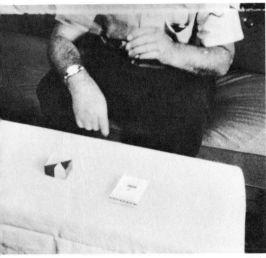

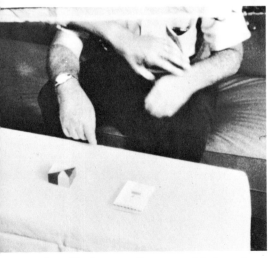

A conflict between disconnected halves of the brain of an epilepsy sufferer is caught in this sequence. Using right hand and left brain—clumsy with spatial relationships—the patient tries vainly to arrange blocks to match a drawing (top). Frustrated, his more adept right brain and left hand, although forbidden to help, try to take over (center) and have to be restrained (bottom).

not understand it and thus was unable to order the hand to follow instructions. Similarly, the subject could not name or describe common objects placed in his left hand if they were hidden from view behind a screen; the sensations of touch had gone to his mute right brain. He might call a pencil a can opener or a cigarette lighter. It was as if the scientists had handed the object to a person in one room, then asked a second person in another room to identify it. When the patient was asked about the activities of his left hand, his responses were also bizarre. Both his brains could hear but only the talking left brain could answer.

It had received no information of the left hand's activities, and therefore replied that it did not remember a thing. In trial after trial, neither hand—and neither brain—knew what the other was doing.

Though the right brain proved greatly inferior to the left brain linguistically, it did not turn out to be completely illiterate. Its capacity varied from one patient to the next. Some of the split-brain patients understood simple words that were flashed to the right brain. In one visual test, for example, the word "heart" was flashed onto the board in front of patients so that only part of the word was accessible to each visual field and thus to each brain. The right brain saw "he." The left brain saw "art." Asked to name the word, the subject's left brain naturally answered "art." But then the mute right brain was given a chance to respond in another way. The subject was given a choice of two printed cards—one with the word "art," the other with "he"—and told to point to the correct one with his left hand. The subjects invariably pointed to "he." The right brain not only observed the portion of the word that lay in its visual field, but it recognized what it saw and could order an appropriate response. This nonverbal brain responded through its own body language.

The right brain also demonstrated the ability to comprehend words when they were spoken. Unlike touch, hearing communicates with both hemispheres. When test subjects were asked to retrieve objects from a hidden grab bag with their left hands, they could pick out the appropriate object—a watch, spoon or comb. They could also do this when the object they were supposed to select was not named but described. For example, if asked to "retrieve the fruit monkeys like best," the left hand promptly pulled a banana from a hidden bag of plastic fruit. But the subjects, though they identified the banana by shape, were unable to give it a name.

The right brain was also proved to possess some other intellectual talents. It could add up to 10. It even demonstrated a rudimentary ability to reason. The right brain was presented with a picture of a cigarette

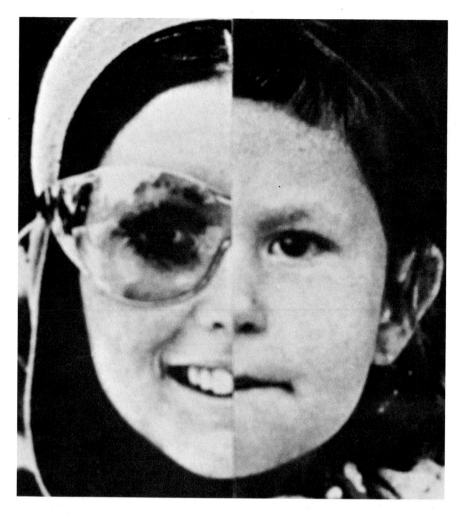

and then the subject was told to select with his left hand the matching item from a hidden assortment of objects. Though the assortment did not actually include a cigarette, the left hand came up with the nearest thing available—an ash tray.

At certain tasks the right brain proved to be superior to its literate counterpart on the left. It controlled the left hand in spatial skills such as arranging blocks to match a pictured design and drawing a cube in three dimensions—but could not copy a written word. The right hand, though retaining its ability to write, could not cope with certain spatial tasks. One subject was unable to copy a simple square with his right hand. He readily drew the four corners but could not link them together with four lines.

Most extraordinary, each brain proved to have a will and emotions of its own. Often, the test situations resembled those occasions, familiar to everyone, when body language speaks louder than words—when gestures and facial expression belie speech and reveal true feelings. In sit-

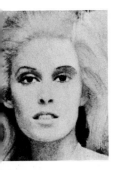
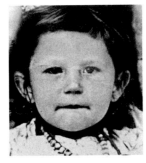
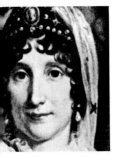
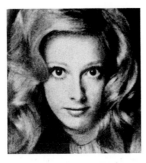
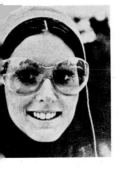
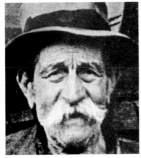

The composite picture at left is used to test split-brain patients—those lacking the normal connection between the two brain halves. Each of the separated brains perceives a different image: the right brain sees the left half of the picture, the left brain sees the right half. When the patient is asked which face from the above group he has seen, his verbal left brain leads him to reply, "the child" (top right, above). But when he is asked to point, his spatial right brain leads him to indicate the woman at bottom left.

uations where only the right brain knew what the left hand was doing, the left brain would make wild guesses. The right brain would then attempt to correct the guesses—by making the face frown or wince or even by shaking the head negatively.

In one of these experiments, the split-brain emotional responses of a young housewife were tested. A picture of a nude woman was flashed to her left hemisphere. She laughed and had no trouble identifying the picture. But when the picture was shown only to her right hemisphere, she could not say what it was. At first she flushed and began squirming. The right brain could not describe the picture, but it reacted emotionally nonetheless. Finally, she broke into a grin and began chuckling. Pressed for an explanation, she responded lamely, "I don't know . . . nothing . . . oh—that funny machine."

The potential for conflict between hemispheres of the split brain is great. There are times when they are at war with themselves, and then the left hand acts as if it does not know what the right hand is doing. This was dramatically illustrated in the travails of one split-brain subject, the war veteran whose brain had been injured by bomb fragments. He possessed above-average intelligence and a good sense of humor. Yet for a short time after surgery he had such quarrelsome hands that sometimes he would attempt to pull up his pants with one while pulling them down with the other.

During one test, he was asked to arrange colored blocks according to a diagram. He could see the blocks and the diagram with both eyes and both brains; thus both brains perceived the problem and could observe the solution. But carrying out the solution involved only one hand and one brain at a time. His left hand, controlled by the spatially gifted right brain, quickly accomplished the task. His right hand, however, fumbled helplessly with the blocks. The left hand then became so persistent in trying to take over the task that the subject had to sit on it. When he attempted the task with both hands, it was even worse. The two hands battled for control, the less skillful left brain commanding the right hand to tear down the work of the other brain and hand. On one occasion he became upset with his wife. He grabbed her with his left hand and shook her while his right hand came to her aid and tried to push the left hand away from her.

The split-brain work and other recent clinical evidence have provided fascinating new portraits of man's two minds. The left brain emerges from these studies as logical, verbal, talented in such subjects as mathematics and science, which require sequential processing of information. The right brain is intuitive, nonverbal, more aware of the body's

The left hand versus the right

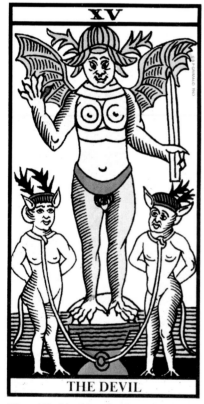

The addled-looking devil pictured on a tarot card used in fortunetelling holds his sword in his left hand or claw. Tarot designs are little changed since Medieval times, when the left hand was thought evil.

That notable American philosopher and dean of baseball-team managers, Casey Stengel, himself a left-hander, once came out strongly if rather elliptically in favor of lefties. "Left-handers have much more enthusiasm for life," Stengel said. "They sleep on the wrong side of the bed, and their heads become stagnant on that side."

If Stengel's conclusion is a trifle murky, that is nothing new; most of what has been said over the ages about left-handedness has made little sense. For countless centuries the left hand was considered cursed or unclean. A number of religions either forbid eating with the left hand or prescribe ritual washings to cleanse the offending member. The Bible, as well as Christian doctrine, is filled with this odd, ancient prejudice. Christ, of course, "sits at the right hand of God the Father almighty." On judgment day the sinners bound for hell will line up on Christ's left. In religious art Christ is invariably pictured using His right hand to bless. Pictures of the devil, by contrast, show him wielding his sword or chivying sinners with his left hand. During the witch trials of the 17th Century, the fact that the accused was left-handed was frequently taken as proof that she was in league with Old Nick and deserved burning.

Such irrational prejudice made left-handers (at most 10 per cent of the world's population) feel like outcasts. Into this century parents of a left-handed child often hid the fact from the neighbors and frequently forced the child to do things right-handed. Similar strong feelings continue in Japan, among other countries. Until recently Japanese school teachers commonly beat left-handed pupils to make them write right-handed and many Japanese girls still pretend to be right-handed in order to get married. If the husband discovers the subterfuge after marriage, the secret lefty may find herself divorced.

Such ancient prejudices have vanished in many countries of the world, partly because parents have been reassured that a left-handed child is not a freak—and warned that attempts to change this natural preference subject the child to psychological harm. Nervous tics, stuttering and trouble in reading and writing have been blamed on misguided efforts to force a child to favor his right hand.

Although there is plenty of evidence that a child should be encouraged to use the hand he chooses, the reasons why such freedom of choice is advisable have proved elusive. For some years scientists placed the responsibility for right- and left-handedness on the division of duties between the twin halves of the brain. Since the left lobe of the brain controls the right side of the body, and the right lobe controls the left, the right lobe was assumed to be dominant for left-handers. So, the theory went, trying to convert a lefty into a righty would hopelessly cross wires in the child's head.

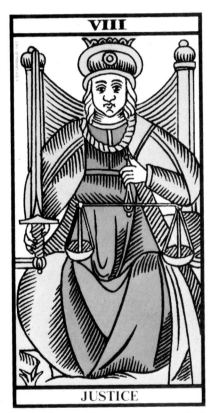

The figure of Justice in the tarot deck holds her sword in her right hand while dangling the scales of justice from her left. According to ancient superstition, the right hand was divinely favored to scourge evil.

This simple explanation now seems inadequate. Oliver L. Zangwill of England's Cambridge University, a leading modern expert on the subject of left-handedness, has found that the right hemisphere of the brain is by no means dominant in all left-handers. More than 50 per cent of the lefties have dominant left brain lobes.

Zangwill also found that many people who write left-handed do other things, such as throwing a ball, right-handed. Right-handers less frequently show such ambidextral tendencies.

These facts led Zangwill to suggest that many left-handers may have ambidextrous brains with neither lobe as dominant as the left lobe is in right-handers. Thus their language ability and kindred processes like writing are not firmly lodged in one lobe of the brain. Lacking a firm left-to-right orientation, left-handers sometimes have difficulty learning to read and write; many try to read right to left and mentally reverse easily reversed letters like "b" and "d."

In addition, Zangwill says, people with ambidextral cerebral organization appear to be particularly vulnerable to stress. This extra sensitivity explains why forcing a left-handed child to become right-handed is dangerous to psychological balance. It is not that wires are being crossed in the head, Zangwill believes, but simply that trying to make a righty out of a lefty produces stress in a child already vulnerable to it.

With the change in popular attitude toward the left-handed have come several mundane but significant improvements in their lot. Until now they have had to cope as best they could in a world made for the right-handed. All sorts of things from corkscrews to school desks have been designed for righties; no culture has ever seen a left-handed scythe or sickle. But today the needs of the lefties are recognized—and served. Shops in London and New York have prospered stocking goods made specially for lefties—nail clippers, pruning shears and pump-action shotguns that eject the empty shells leftward instead of past the left-handed shooter's nose.

Even while left-handers often suffered the inconvenience of making do with wrong-handed implements, they profited from certain natural advantages. Other experts besides Casey Stengel agree that the left-handed have an extra measure of zest; and if they seem to be less logical than staid righties, they are believed to possess richer stores of creativity. After all, using the left hand hardly seems to have cramped the style of Charlemagne, Leonardo da Vinci or Ben Franklin. And baseball fans have long known the curious advantage that helped Casey Stengel get his start in the sport. The layout of the baseball diamond gives left-handed batters a special benefit: they are nearer first base when they stand at the plate and have a shorter distance to run after a hit.

orientation in space. Another distinctive feature of the right brain is its musical ability. Tests with victims of strokes and other disorders have indicated that damage to the right brain often wipes out the capacity to recognize differences in musical sounds. On the other hand, in one striking case a Russian composer who suffered a stroke in his left brain, and was unable to comprehend the verbal sounds of speech, continued to be able to distinguish between intervals of musical sound, and went on writing wonderful symphonies.

The new appreciation of the right brain is one of the most surprising results of split-brain research. Even in its weakest talent, language, the right brain shows unexpected potential. Apparently its muteness is not ordained by evolution but develops only relatively late in childhood. One striking confirmation of the right brain's language potential is the case of an 11-year-old boy who had been born without any corpus callosum at all. Tests showed that each of his brains had developed and retained full capacity for language. That a fragment of this ability survives in adults is indicated not only by the split-brain experiments but also by several instances from medical history. There is, for example, a case in which language ability survived in a 47-year-old man whose entire left hemisphere was surgically removed because of a tumor. The man woke up from the operation cursing and soon was able to communicate his thoughts in short, halting phrases. He even learned to print words with his left hand.

These observations, buttressed by the results of split-brain research, have led Michael Gazzaniga to propose methods for rehabilitating victims of brain damage. He points out that when the right brain of a split-brain subject was presented with the printed word "pencil," the left hand was able to find one in a bag of hidden objects. It seemed able to respond to simple nouns, although not to verbs like "smile" or "laugh." One patient, by arranging plastic letters with his left hand, managed to spell out nouns such as "pie" and "cup."

Such latent capacities of the right brain might enable stroke victims, many of whom are deprived of verbal ability by damage to the left brain, to learn to carry on rudimentary communication with their right brains. One medium, Gazzaniga suggests, could be symbols of the kind that have proved successful in the "talking ape" experiments. Plastic symbols have been used to teach chimpanzees to comprehend a few words and even to construct some sentences. One of Gazzaniga's graduate students used cutout symbols made of construction paper to help stroke victims who could not speak or understand speech. She found that she was able to teach these people to spell out such words as "same" and "different" with their left hands and even to arrange the symbols into simple statements.

The philosophical implications of the split-brain research are even more intriguing. The results provide a physiological explanation for an old and familiar observation about human behavior. There long have appeared to be two different ways of thinking: some people are essentially verbal and analytical, while others are nonverbal and intuitive. These two ways of thinking coincide neatly with the concept of two brains, the analytical left hemisphere and the intuitive right hemisphere.

In Western societies, the emphasis on rational thought that began in the Renaissance has for centuries favored the left brain at the expense of the irrational right brain. And yet man's highest achievements seem to stem from the successful integration of both left-brain intellect and right-brain intuition. This is true even in science, where the primary emphasis—at least in the development of a scientific idea—is on rational, linear thinking.

Nearly all discoveries in every field appear to involve a sudden right-brain inspiration. At an idle moment, maybe even in a dream, intuition makes an intellectual leap—sensing a solution to a long-standing problem, arriving at fresh understanding, reaching a new level of appreciation—in one quick burst of illumination. Then the left-brain intellect laboriously works out the details of this hunch, step by step. Without the left brain's patient attention to detail, the right-brain hunch may remain fantasy. One of the most brilliant thinkers of modern times, Albert Einstein, once remarked that his first inkling of a new idea often came to him by intuition—sometimes in visual images. "The really valuable thing is intuition," Einstein said. "A thought comes and I may try to express it in words afterwards."

Einstein's statement encapsulates the crucial role of each brain in the creative process. Without the right brain, there would be no idea; without the left brain, the idea could not be explained. Now split-brain research has provided scientists with an unprecedented opportunity to explore the reality behind statements like the one made by Einstein.

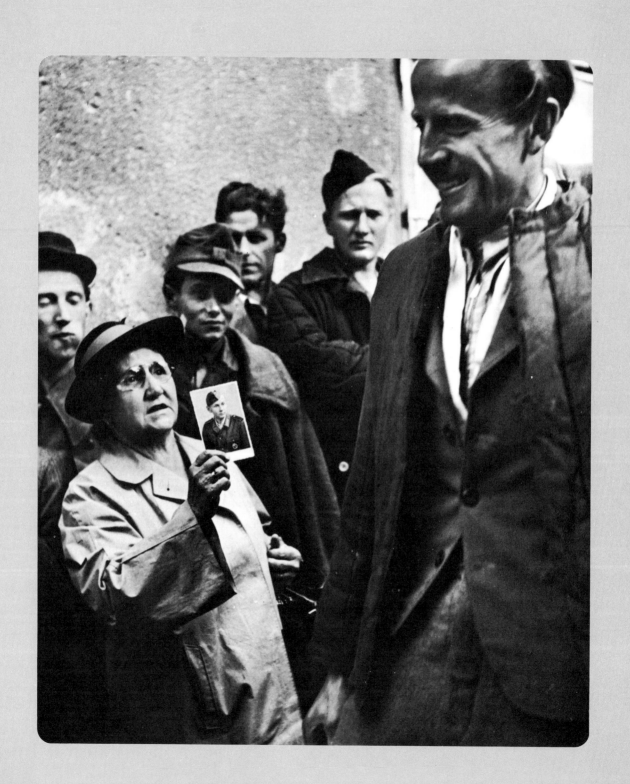

The Mystery of Memory

George and Charles are identical twins, and both are mentally retarded. At age 26 their IQs, in the range of 60 to 70, gave them intelligence equivalent to that of an eight- or 10-year-old child. Yet George and Charles could perform phenomenal feats of memory. When asked, "In what months of the year 2002 does the first of the month fall on a Friday?" George replied without a moment's hesitation: "In March, February and November." "When does April 21 fall on a Sunday?" continued the questioner, and quick as a flash the answer came back, "In 1968, 1957, 1963, 1946. . . ."

George and Charles are idiot savants, a term probably coined by French scholars who were among the first to study the occasionally astonishing memory skills demonstrated by the feeble-minded. There are dozens of case histories of people like George and Charles, but the twins are probably the most famous. As residents of the New York State Psychiatric Institute, their peculiar talents were closely studied.

Like many idiot savants, George and Charles focused their peculiar gifts on mathematical problems, specifically on calendrical calculations. With almost unerring accuracy they could tell on what particular day of the week a particular date would fall, and they did so for dates ranging all the way from 4,100 B.C. to 40,400 A.D. No one knows how they performed their lightning calculations. Formerly it was assumed that idiot savants memorized material by rote learning, and they were presumed able to do so because their minds were incapable of doing much else. They did it superbly well. But there were no calendars for George and Charles to memorize for many of the centuries they dealt with. Clearly, they must have had some system of computation that depended on memory. Yet their memory for other mathematical data was so limited that they could not even memorize the multiplication table. Asked what seven times four meant, one replied, "It means 14."

How idiot savants remember and why they remember only certain kinds of information is a puzzle that may never be solved. The whole field of memory is one that continues to perplex scientists. Theories about it abound, however, some of them so intriguing that they make newspaper headlines. It has been suggested, for instance, that the memory areas of the brain are transferable from one body to another, like transplanted kidneys. It has even been suggested that memory tissue can be chopped up and served like a dietary supplement, to provide instant learning. Behind the spectacular headlines, scientists are quietly accumulating clues that may eventually solve the puzzle of memory. Already it is clear that there are several different kinds of memory, that they operate differently and that they may be in different locations.

Some of the clues being followed by memory scientists are easily discerned by anyone who taxes his own memory about how he remembers. He quickly realizes that his visual memory, recalling images, is quite distinct from his verbal memory, for words and language. And the memories stored as pictures tend to be the stronger of these two types. In a story by Argentinian writer Jorge Luis Borges, a man named Funes the Memorious remembered "the shape of the clouds in the south at dawn on the 30th of April of 1882, and he could compare them in his recollection with the marbled grain in the design of a leather-bound book which he has seen only once, and with the lines in the spray which an oar raised in the Rio Negro on the eve of the battle of Quebracho."

The power of the visual memory may account for the remarkable phenomenon of the photographic memory possessed by many children. Technically known as eidetic memory, it allows them to summon up in their minds a detailed image of something they want to remember. When trying to recall a historical fact or the spelling of a word, they create a mental picture of the necessary page in the textbook and simply read off what they need to know. This valuable power rarely survives puberty. Apparently some selection process takes over as the brain matures, and makes memory more discriminating. Instead of remembering a whole printed page, the brain remembers only the relevant words and tosses out the rest. Perhaps the indiscriminate eidetic memory of childhood explains why the remembrances of early years are often so full of detail. They are cluttered with the charming minutiae that more discerning adult minds screen out as unworthy of keeping.

The division between visual and verbal memories is paralleled by another fundamental and obvious distinction in types of memory, one based on the length of time something is remembered. Casual observation and careful experiments both show that some memories are short-term and others long-term. Short-term memories disappear in a half-hour or so, and are often called telephone-number memories because the digits of a telephone number generally linger in the mind only long enough to dial them. Long-term memories appear to remain on call for a lifetime. They become so firmly established in the brain's complex file of thoughts and sensations that most are capable of surviving electric shock, drugs, sometimes even amnesia.

The duration of a memory is partly determined by the importance of the material being remembered. Since the events remembered best and longest are those with the highest emotional charge, some scientists think the brain's emotional centers help determine which memories are short, which long. The key element, they believe, is the hippocampus, a small curved chunk of gray matter, a little more than an inch long, that is tucked under the temporal lobe on each side of the head. Its function seems to resemble that of the "now print" button on a computer. Taking its cues from emotional centers nearby, the hippocampus impresses the details of an emotion-packed event on the memory circuits.

Damage to the hippocampus appears to render the brain incapable of long-term memories. The most notable case history of this condition is a man known in medical literature simply as H. M. In 1953, surgery on H. M.'s temporal lobes to relieve severe epilepsy inadvertently damaged his hippocampus and robbed him of the ability to remember. Though H. M. retained all the memories that had been stored before his operation, he could remember almost nothing new. Nothing seemed to stick in his mind much over 15 minutes. Every time he visited his doctors, they had to reintroduce themselves, and he read the same issue of a magazine over and over without realizing he had seen it before.

But H. M.'s lack of memory was not entirely consistent. "In spells," as his mother put it, he made a new memory. In the late 1960s, he recognized the likeness of John F. Kennedy on a coin and remembered the former President's assassination, an event that had occurred nearly a decade after H. M.'s operation. Apparently the emotional impact of that tragedy was so overwhelming that it generated an electrical impulse powerful enough to sweep through his damaged hippocampus and set off the now-print button. Indeed, most people above a certain age can remember the Kennedy assassination—and the public events surrounding it—with extraordinary clarity. Many vividly recall where they were when they heard the news, and exactly what they were doing. Obviously some events burn themselves into the memory simply and purely from the intensity of the emotional charge that accompanies them.

The fact that the emotional centers and the hippocampus seem to have some bearing on memory does not necessarily mean that they are

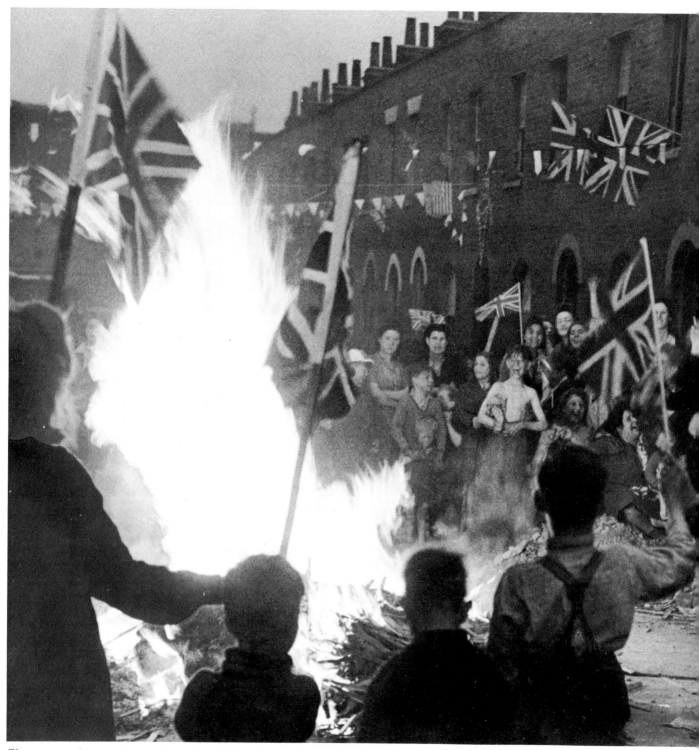

The memory of an emotionally charged experience like this London bonfire celebration of Allied victory in Europe in 1945 often lasts a lifetime. The event becomes permanent, perhaps by capturing brain circuits and occupying them long enough to make an ineradicable record.

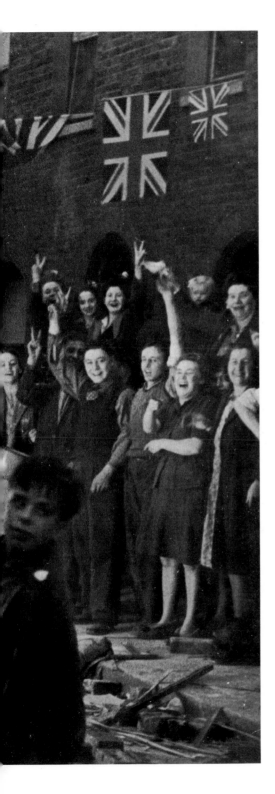

where memory resides. Scientists in fact do not know the locale of memory. However, the visual and verbal types of memory do seem to be associated with particular parts of the brain, leading many scientists to believe that all memories may someday be localized. This belief is nurtured by the widely held assumption that memory is somehow encoded in the labyrinthine nerve circuits of the brain. If so, the coded material must logically be stored according to some sort of grand scheme. The search for such a scheme has been long and discouraging, but the elements of it are at last being detected.

One of the first men to seek memory's elusive locale was the American neuro-psychologist Karl Lashley. Beginning in the 1920s, Lashley spent nearly three decades looking for the physical traces of memory. He taught rats to find their way through mazes and then surgically removed various parts of their brain surfaces in order to pinpoint the source of their maze-running skill. To his surprise, no single area of the cortex seemed to contain the wiring for this newly acquired aptitude. Though removal of a brain section always canceled out some maze training, the loss was one of degree—the more cortex Lashley cut away, the greater the loss of memory. Also, no matter where Lashley cut, the rats always managed somehow to limp, roll or stagger through the maze. Thus, instead of being localized, memory was apparently everywhere.

At the very time Lashley was sadly concluding that memory had no physical existence, a Canadian neurosurgeon, Wilder Penfield, was stumbling upon a curious phenomenon suggesting that it did. Penfield, a specialist in surgery to relieve epilepsy, focused his attention on the tiny area of scar tissue from which epileptic seizures start, spreading their fire storm of electrical signals through the brain. To locate this critical area he used an electrical probe, passing it over the surface of the brain to stimulate various parts. The patient, though conscious, felt no pain and described the resulting sensations. When the probe passed over the vision center, the patient reported seeing bursts of light or kaleidescopic colors; when it passed over the area concerned with hearing, it activated buzzing sounds or musical tones.

During the course of one such exploratory operation in 1936, Penfield discovered that his probe could provoke full-blown memories. The memories were described by his patients as if they were scenes from a movie; the patient was a passive spectator rather than an active participant. "Oh, gosh!" exclaimed one 12-year-old boy, "There they are, my brother is there. He is aiming an air rifle at me." A young woman relived a concert and hummed along with the music the orchestra was playing. A young man saw the South African farm he had come from.

All of the memories played back in Penfield's operating room had one thing in common: Each resulted from stimulation of the same general region of the brain, the region next to the ear and temple known as the temporal lobe, and Penfield concluded that the lobe holds at least part of the circuitry of memory. Not all other brain researchers agree with him. The brains of epileptics, they point out, have an abnormal electrical activity, making it difficult to pinpoint the actual area being affected by the electrode. Besides, when the temporal lobes of normal people are stimulated, no movie-scene memories appear.

Nevertheless, there is some support for Penfield's premise. From the evidence of two experiments conducted at Princeton and Stanford universities on monkeys, it appears that one type of memory, visual memory, is indeed stored in the temporal lobes. In the Princeton studies, psychologist Charles Gross and his colleagues have found that one group of nerve cells in a monkey's temporal lobe fires with particular intensity when the monkey sees a pattern resembling the shape of its hand, a shape so familiar that it would naturally be easily remembered. In somewhat similar research at Stanford, psychologist K. L. Chow discovered that when a monkey's temporal nerve cells were damaged, the animal could not retain visual skills previously acquired and could not learn new ones—apparently because the mechanism for storing visual memories had been impaired.

Such glimpses into the possible locale of memory are tantalizing, but they are only a beginning step toward finding the answers to a much larger question: How is memory formed? Two different mechanisms seem likely, one for short memories, one for long.

Telephone-number memories, those that last only a half-hour or so, may consist of electrical activity only. The electrical impulse in a nerve circuit reverberates through the circuit continuously, like an echo lingering in the air of an Alpine valley. When the signal dies out, it disappears without leaving any record of its presence. Such a memory is as ephemeral as an Alpinist's yodel. The fragility of short-term memory supports this theory. Anything that disrupts the transmission of nerve impulses plays hob with short-term memory.

Long-term memories are different. They generally survive all kinds of hardship. Even a blow to the head severe enough to cause amnesia may not destroy them. Although the victim loses all sense of past history in the moments immediately after the traumatic event, the long-term memories ordinarily come back. This evidence suggests that long-term memories are not purely electrical. But how are the fragile electrical impulses of short-term storage converted into a permanent record? Most scientists believe that the repeated electrical firing of short-term memory, if continued long enough, alters the configuration of the nerve circuit—in much the same way that a riverbed is altered by a river that overflows its banks in flood. Such permanent changes would have to be structural and biochemical, and a number of fascinating and controversial theories have attempted to explain how they come about.

If the long-term memory is a structure in the brain—a new circuit or a special substance—the brain cells have to build it. The most likely building material is a protein, one of the broad class of large, complex compounds that make up nearly all living tissue. Nerve cells are known to manufacture and use up more protein than any other kind of cell —so much, in fact, that the average life of a protein molecule in a nerve cell may be as little as a few minutes. This mass protein production must have a reason, and perhaps the reason is memory storage.

Because protein molecules are large and complex, their parts can be arranged in a multitude of ways, and these varied designs can serve as a code, like the alphabet of a language. Different proteins become different "words," each with its own meaning. There could easily be enough distinct proteins to account for the structural changes involved in storing the 100 trillion bits of memory accumulated in a lifetime.

Evidence for the role of proteins in memory comes from experiments showing stepped-up protein production in rats and chickens during various learning experiments. Holger Hydén, Director of the Institute of Neurobiology at the University of Göteborg in Sweden, found that rats trained to climb a rope increased their output of RNA, a substance necessary to the manufacture of protein, during the training period. He also found that two specific kinds of protein appeared in the rats' brains during this same period. At Britain's Open University, biochemist Steven Rose charted the instinctive process by which a baby chick learns to recognize its mother and noted a buildup of both protein and RNA in the chick's brain during the mother-recognition process.

Working from the opposite tack, other researchers have found evidence of change in the learning process when protein production is blocked. At the University of Michigan, for instance, Bernard Agranoff conducted a series of experiments on fish, creatures that, as any fisherman knows, have long memories. Agranoff taught goldfish to swim the length of a fish tank whenever a light flashed on, a skill the fish ordinarily remembered for at least a month. But if he injected a drug that interferes with protein manufacture, puromycin, into the fish's brain immediately before or after the training session, the fish could not remember its swimming task. On the other hand, if the puromycin was injected an hour after the lesson was over, the fish's memory was not affected—apparently because the necessary protein had been made and the lesson had already been implanted.

While most scientists agree that protein production is somehow involved in long-term memory storage, a few go well beyond this orthodox view. They suggest that protein molecules themselves are storage containers for memory. This idea has nourished the intriguing notion that an entire memory—say, the score of Beethoven's Fifth Symphony —might be encoded in a single protein molecule. Such extreme suppositions have led to a whole series of serious but controversial studies. If memories are embedded in brain molecules it would seem possible to train an animal to perform an unfamiliar task and then graft pieces of its brain onto an untrained animal to transfer the skill; the second animal would acquire knowledge by injection. A number of scientists have tried to do just that.

The first of the "memory molecule" experiments were carried out in the early 1960s by James McConnell at the University of Michigan. McConnell is a rather flamboyant psychologist who was working at the time with tiny flatworms and on the side editing a partly humorous scientific journal, *Worm-Runner's Digest*. McConnell trained tiny flatworms to respond to light, and then tried to implant this skill in untrained worms by grafting. Unfortunately most of his worms died. Then he took the more direct route of chopping up the trained worms and feeding tiny chunks of them to their untrained brethren. This procedure, McConnell reported, was a success—a conclusion that brought newspaper headlines and raised eyebrows throughout the scientific community. But the work of one of McConnell's associates provoked even greater controversy. In 1965, Allan Jacobson announced that he had transferred learning in rats by extracting the protein-making substance, RNA, from the brains of trained rats and injecting it into untrained ones. Later that year, in an unusual step, 23 scientists wrote to the magazine *Science* announcing that none had been able to duplicate the experiment.

Discouraged by the skeptical reception their ideas received, McConnell and Jacobson gave up their memory molecule research, and in later years its only active proponent was Georges Ungar, Professor of Pharmacology at Baylor College of Medicine in Houston, Texas. Ungar reported that he had transferred learned behavior from one mouse brain to another by extracting the protein molecule in which one kind of new learning is embedded. The acquired learning was fear of the dark (chosen for study because it is unnatural behavior in mice), and Ungar

continued on page 105

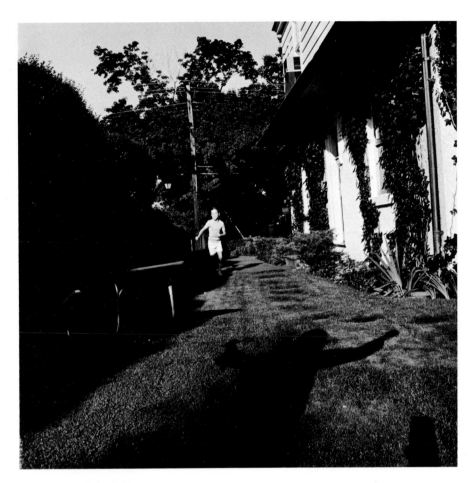

In the backyard of her Aunt Marion's house in Port Washington, New York, Melissa Shook's shadow looms in the foreground as she photographs her daughter Krissy racing toward the camera. Although Melissa often played in this yard when she was Krissy's age, amnesia has clouded her memory of it.

A childhood lost to amnesia

The key events in most people's lives become so deeply embedded in memory that they survive every hardship. But in rare instances, extremely painful or emotionally charged experiences can partially or completely cancel memory. Such a poignant loss was suffered by New York photographer Melissa Shook, whose mother died when Melissa was 12. The experience was so shattering that it left her with partial amnesia. For more than 20 years, she had only a fragmentary memory of the event and the years that preceded it.

The feeling of loss and insecurity bothered Melissa so much that, when she was 33 years old, she decided to confront the emotion-laden scenes of her childhood and try to put the experience into proper focus. Because the house where she had grown up had been sold long ago, she visited her aunt, who was especially close to her mother, and in whose house Melissa had spent a lot of time as a child. She took a camera with her, setting it up to photograph herself in the once-familiar surroundings, as a way of trying to resolve the emotional trauma and sort out the fragments of her lost memories.

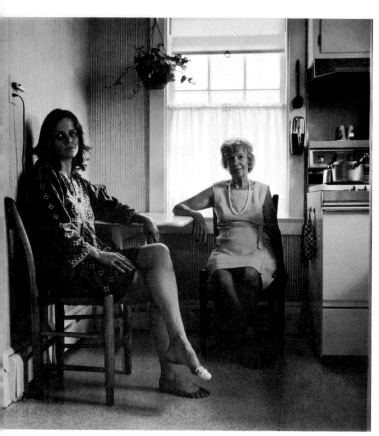

In the kitchen of the Port Washington, New York, house, Melissa photographs herself and her aunt. "My aunt's home is the closest I can come to the familiarity of those early years," Melissa says, "and my Aunt Marion is my closest link to my real mother."

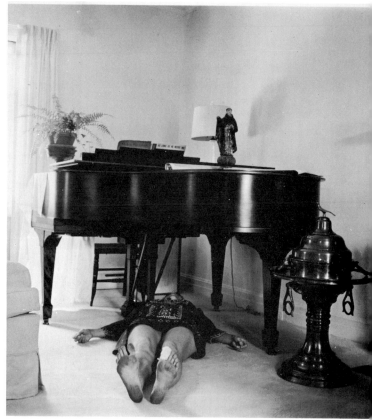

Melissa stretches out under her aunt's piano—where her father and uncle used to lie down and take naps on the floor after big holiday meals.

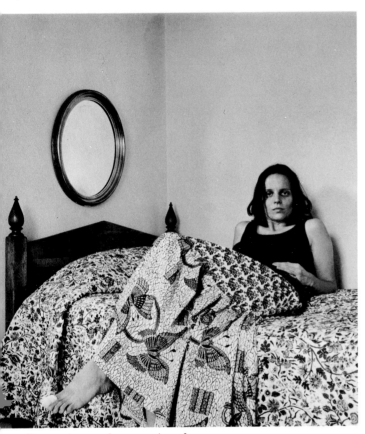

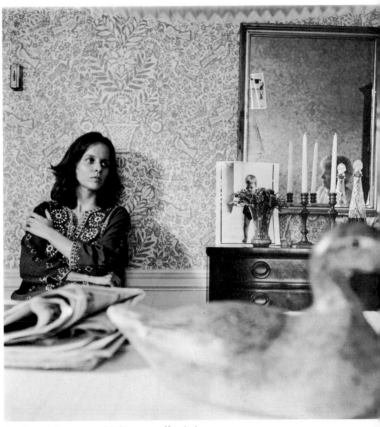

Re-creating another scene from her childhood, Melissa rests on a bed where she remembers her cousin lying one day. The mirror on the wall may be one that her mother bought, she conjectures, but she is not really sure.

In the dining room, Melissa recalls sitting at the table at Thanksgiving or Christmas and seeing herself in the mirror just as her aunt is reflected here.

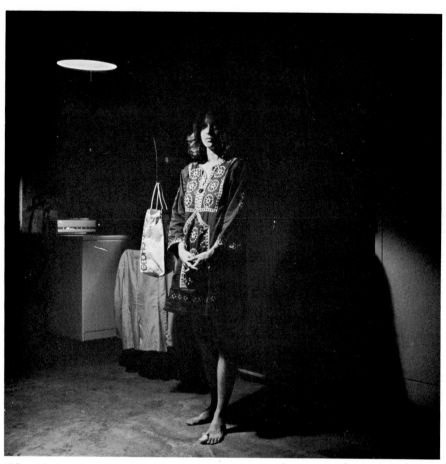

A haunting memory comes back as Melissa visits the basement of her aunt's home. "The open-backed stairs down to my aunt's cellar frightened me when I was a child," she says; "I remember that fear, and sometimes I dream about the basement now." Melissa found that her visit to her aunt enabled her to conquer some of her anxiety but thinks now that the missing memories will never return. Psychologists supply the reason why this may be so. They say that people may suppress a painful memory because, unconsciously, they want to forget it.

claimed he had synthesized the molecule responsible. He called this memory molecule scotophobin, from the Greek for fear of darkness. Most scientists, however, remain doubtful about Ungar's results and the conclusions have been challenged in the journals even more strongly than Jacobson's. The skeptics point out that a molecule like scotophobin seems too heavy to serve as a memory storage unit. If the remembrances of the average human were encoded in molecules of this size, his memories alone would weigh in the neighborhood of 200 pounds.

Even if memory by injection is not around the corner, other possible consequences of a link between memory and protein production may be almost as startling. Drugs might enhance protein production, and thus improve a person's ability to learn and remember. Scientists have long known that certain drugs speed up the learning process in laboratory animals by making them more alert. Minute quantities of the poison strychnine have been fed to rats for this purpose, for instance, and so has amphetamine, the stimulant familiarly known as speed. Now new drugs are being developed specifically to accelerate the production of protein in humans. One, pemoline, was tested on medical students to see if it helped them learn faster; in another experiment, massive doses of synthetic RNA were fed to elderly people to see if it improved their memories. But such tests are inconclusive, and few scientists expect quick development of chemicals to aid learning and remembering.

The most useful answers to the riddle of memory may come from slowly gathering, bit by bit, clues to the chemical and electrical processes involved in remembering and forgetting. This work involves a painstaking cell-by-cell search through the primitive brains of the simplest creatures, and like Karl Lashley's original search for the source of the maze-running skill of rats, it is concerned with the circuitry that triggers behavior. One of the favorite creatures for this research is the giant sea slug *aplysia*, which grows to about a foot in length and has relatively few but quite large nerve cells—up to 1/25 of an inch in diameter—enabling scientists to tap into them with microelectrodes, record their electrical activity and chart their simple wiring plans.

From studies of the *aplysia's* nerve cell activities, New York physiologist Eric Kandel has made some important discoveries about two elementary forms of learning, habituation and dishabituation. Habituation is learning to ignore a stimulus that has lost its novelty. Humans learn to ignore, for instance, the sensation of a freshly starched shirt rubbing against the skin when they first get dressed in the morning. Similarly, *aplysia* can habituate themselves to ordinarily disturbing sensory signals. When one of these animals is touched near its gill, the gill will normally retract into a cavity for self-protection. But if the gill is stimulated repeatedly, it will eventually stop retracting—a case of the sensory circuits crying "Wolf!" too often.

Dishabituation is the opposite of this kind of learning. It is learning *not* to ignore a repeated stimulus. An *aplysia* that is given an electric shock near its gill twice a day for a number of days running will become so sensitized that it overreacts. The merest touch—a touch far below the normal threshhold of response—will be enough to send the gill into spasms of retraction.

Kandel's experiments with these two kinds of behavior were elegantly simple. First he inserted microelectrodes in the *aplysia's* abdomen near the nerve circuits for the gill. Then he taught the *aplysia* to become habituated to being touched and, afterward, dishabituated. In both cases he recorded the firing pattern of the nerve cells, and in both cases he found that the nerve cell's electrical activity paralleled the animal's behavior. During habituation, electrical activity decreased until finally the cells ceased firing altogether; during dishabituation, they fired repeatedly and intensely. Kandel decided these changes were related to variations in the amount of transmitter chemical released by the cells —the means by which a nerve signal is propelled across the synaptic gap between nerve cells *(Chapter 2)*. And he concluded that in the *aplysia* at least, the newly learned behavioral patterns are programmed into the synapses connecting those nerve cells. Presumably, some physical change alters the mechanism for producing or releasing the transmitter. This change is, in effect, a memory.

Whether humans remember the same way sea slugs do, by remodeling their synapses, no one knows. If they do, the physical trace of memory will have been found in a slight but crucial alteration of nerve endings. But this is only the memory code, the recording system. The major mystery remains: the playback system of recall. How does the mind summon up the data encoded and stored in its memory circuits? Recall, at the cellular level, is a total mystery. It can be triggered by will or by chance and, once in motion, it instantaneously searches the maze of wiring, matching and comparing the stimulus against the billions of coded memory patterns until it finds the appropriate recollection. In special circumstances it can dredge up memories an individual did not even know he had. In dreams, under hypnosis or when influenced by "truth drugs" such as Sodium Pentothal, people sometimes remember scenes from their past lives in the most vivid and minute detail. One bricklayer, under hypnosis, was able to describe every bump and grain on the surface of a brick wall he had laid 20 years before.

The study of recall abounds with such implausible anecdotes—and with a multitude of unanswered questions. Why is it impossible to remember infancy? Perhaps it is because infant memories are stored before the faculty of speech is acquired, and thus cannot be recalled in verbal form—although they may still be implanted in the brain, unconsciously influencing adult behavior. Why do old people have trouble remembering recent events, and yet recall their youth with greater clarity than at any other time in their lives? More baffling still is the enigmatic way in which the mechanism of recall can be turned on by the slightest stimulus. The trigger of a single word, a bar of music, an image, can set off a whole train of memories.

Just as mysterious as the mechanics of recall are those of its opposite: the unjustly maligned process of forgetting. Although the ability to recall is much admired, the ability to forget is equally important. Obviously the mind would collapse if it were required to find room for every potential memory. Apparently the mechanisms of forgetting exist at several stages of the memory-forming process. To begin with, the brain blots out millions of bits of incoming memory material every minute of the day. This perceptual filtering enables the brain to pay attention, to stay in focus, by screening out the myriad impressions constantly assaulting the senses. At a crowded cocktail party, for instance, perceptual filtering sifts through the babel of voices and swirl of faces and eliminates most of them, so that they never reach the brain's center of awareness. Short-term memory also evaluates incoming facts and images, and disposes of those unsuitable for permanent storage.

But even when stored permanently, memories can become inaccessible to the process of recall. Sometimes they are overlaid by newer, more significant streams of data with stronger electrical signals. The latter phenomenon is called the interference theory of forgetting, and it is commonly illustrated with a classic anecdote about an absent-minded professor of ichthyology who claimed that every time he memorized the name of a student, he forgot the name of a fish. And sometimes forgotten memories fade with age, like pigment on an old painting.

The fading process accelerates in middle age, as irreplaceable brain cells begin to die off, several thousand every day. Names, facts and faces that once were at the tip of the tongue elude recall. This weakening of the brain's mysterious power to record and play back the events of a lifetime becomes a mark of advancing years, a saddening reminder of mortality. For a man is the sum of his uniquely remembered experiences, and his memory is central to his individual existence.

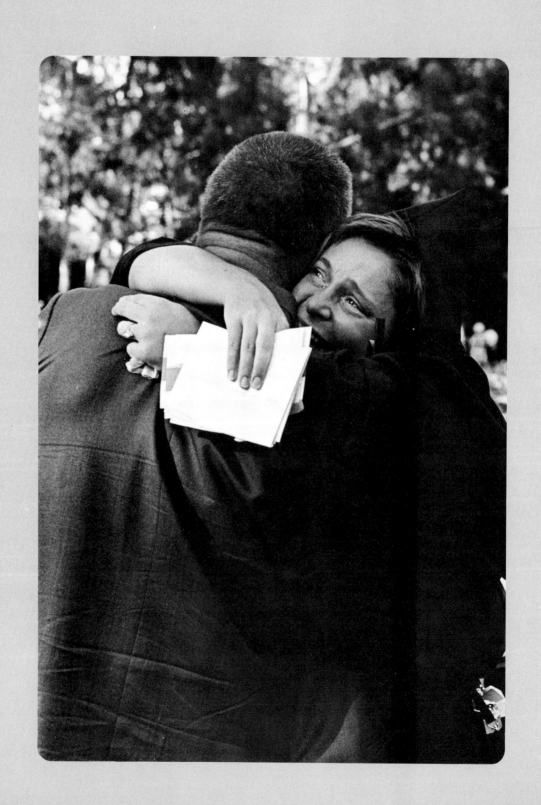

Wellsprings of Feeling

In 1924 in his laboratory in the University of Zurich, Switzerland, Walter R. Hess, eventually to be famous for his exploration of the brain with electric probes, stimulated a cat near the nerve areas he had found to be associated with eating and other bodily functions. He touched a sore spot. The electric current enraged the animal, and it behaved "as if threatened by a dog," Hess reported. In later experiments he observed: "It spits, snorts or growls . . . its pupils widen . . . its ears lie back, or move back and forth to frighten the nonexistent enemy." The cats, normally docile, became so angry under stimulation at a certain point in the brain that one assaulted Hess himself. But stimulation in another spot made the cats cower in fear.

Hess's historic discoveries have now been amplified by other experiments that pinpoint many of the brain mechanisms controlling human feelings. In laboratories throughout the world scientists have been able —by directing chemicals or electric currents to certain areas of the brains of animals and, in special cases, humans—to stimulate a variety of desired instinctual responses in their subjects. They have discovered that it is possible to switch on and off, at will, feelings of love, hate, rage, fear, pleasure and so on. Cats have been made to cower in abject terror in the presence of mice; rats have been rendered ecstatic by electrical stimulation of their deep pleasure centers.

Such experiments are beginning to explain the interactions of feelings and behavior, revealing how electrical and chemical triggers and message carriers, coursing the grids of the brain and nervous system, move an individual from impulse to action. Along with enlightenment, however, comes the specter of possible misuse, for such knowledge may bring the possibility of mind control. It is in the emotion-controlling regions of the brain that scientists have located the once-secret mechanisms determining not just why humans behave like humans, but why one type of human, for instance, may behave and feel like a man and another may behave and feel like a woman, and why, under similar circumstances, one person's response is violent and another's is timid.

The most basic of human feelings are the unlearned instincts, such as hunger, sex, anger, fear, aggression and even pleasure. They have been wired into the brain's circuitry by evolution to ensure physical and psychological well-being. Eating obviously preserves life, sex, the species. Equally important, these drives enable an individual to avoid danger, fight for self-preservation and seek out the pleasures that sustain him. If these feelings are suppressed, the brain and body may answer back with chronic fatigue, ulcers and the various psychosomatic symptoms that in some studies have made up as much as two thirds of all the complaints dealt with by doctors.

Interacting with the primitive drives are equally powerful feelings exhibited in a myriad of automatic emotional responses that are not necessarily instinctual but learned, some directly, some obliquely. Racial discrimination is one good example. Emotional feelings may reinforce a primal drive, or they may countermand it. A resident of the Riviera, bred on seafood, finds delight in satisfying his hunger drive with a dish of raw oysters. In Alsace, far from the ocean, a half-starved man might find the same food so strange he would turn away from it. In neither instance are the oysters responsible for the result. Yet in one case they produce a feeling of pleasure; in the other, aversion.

The basic, instinctual feelings lie, understandably, in a primitive region of the brain—below the bulging cerebral cortex of rational thought so highly prized by man. Here, several interconnected structures at the top of the brain stem form a kind of ring called the limbic system. The ring's major components are the hypothalamus, the amygdala and the hippocampus; of these, the hypothalamus is the most important. Directly, through nerve impulses, or indirectly, through its control of glands that release the behavior-influencing chemicals, hormones, the hypothalamus regulates sex and growth and the responses to hunger, thirst, cold and stress. In the middle of the ring but outside the limbic system is the thalamus, central switchboard for relaying signals between the spinal cord and the brain's surface.

Parts of the limbic system are deeply involved in the sense of smell, and they constitute what is sometimes called the smell brain. In many lower animals smell is the dominant sense, and the brain's drive centers may have developed originally in this region, to provide immediate responses to the most crucial scents—food and the presence of an enemy. Even in man specific odors still evoke basic responses. The aroma of broiling steak can make the mouth water; exotic perfume is designed to stir a man's desire; and there is now some evidence that bodily odors called pheromones influence sexual activity in humans as they are known to do among animals. Thus the centers of instinct not only generate feelings but also contain blueprints for the appropriate behavioral response to a feeling—the action that will satisfy the need.

Most animals automatically act out their prewired rituals of eating, courtship and fighting. In man the large cerebral hemispheres that evolved around and above the instinctual areas, where learned reactions are stored, mediate how he responds to the insistent promptings of an instinctive drive. He can feel angry, hungry or sexually aroused; but ordinarily he can modify his course. He can suppress hunger and refuse a second helping at mealtime, channel an erotic mood onto another track of self-fulfillment or vent his anger on a football field.

The experiments that identified the roles of these brain centers in behavior are among the most spectacular in this field of science. They owe their beginnings to Walter R. Hess not only because he made the initial discoveries but also because he developed the techniques now employed (he was awarded a Nobel Prize in 1949). In place of the previous method of inserting wires for each test—a practice subject to human error —he inserted the electrodes semipermanently, locating them carefully and attaching them to fixed terminals on the animals' scalps. He wired the terminals to instruments hung from the ceiling so that his cats could move about as if on a leash and thus act in a reasonably normal way. Today the terminals can be connected to small radio transmitters, so that the animal subjects move freely, almost as if they were not being studied. With this and other equipment, experimenters have refined and extended the map of the brain's role in emotions and feelings.

Because of the brain's complexity, and the known interrelationship between conscious and unconscious circuits in a wide variety of behavioral responses, many scientists questioned Hess's conclusion that he had located centers of rage and fear. They did not quibble with the fact that his electric current had produced behavior resembling rage and fear. But they suggested that the apparent emotions were sham—a physical acting out, lacking the feeling itself. Such intense emotions as pain and pleasure were believed to involve excitation of the entire brain and thus could not be elicited in any single center of brain tissue. Then, in the early 1950s, two groups of researchers dramatically demonstrated that specific brain centers could give rise to genuine feelings. One feeling was aversion, a feeling so unpleasant that an animal would try desperately to avoid it. The other was pleasure, a feeling so rewarding that the animal would seek it at almost any cost.

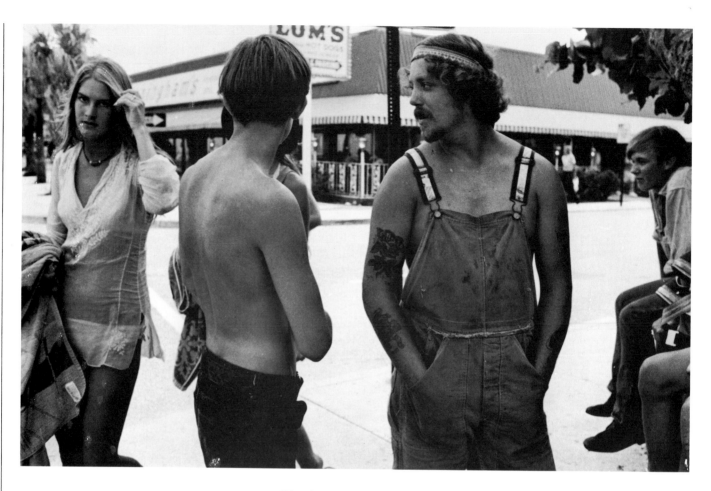

The first group of researchers, at Yale, experimented with cats that had electrodes implanted in several areas just above the hypothalamus. The scientists presented the hungry cats with food, then switched on the current. The cats immediately stopped eating, as if stung by the food. When the experiment was repeated, the cats avoided the food completely despite their hunger. The current itself was not strong enough to shock them severely and similar stimulation in other parts of the brain had only a brief distracting effect. But around the hypothalamus the current had touched clusters of terribly unpleasant nerves, triggering built-in mechanisms of punishment.

Soon after, a young American psychologist working at McGill University in Montreal happened upon even more astonishing sources of intense feeling in the brain. James Olds was attempting to stimulate an area below a rat's hypothalamus, a region known to be involved in sleep and wakefulness. The rat, a pair of wires strung from its head, was free to move about in a table-top enclosure three feet square. Every time the animal entered a particular corner Olds turned on the current. Olds assumed the brief jolt would teach the rat to avoid that corner. To the contrary, the rat kept coming back for more as if the shock had aroused its curiosity. But more than its curiosity was being stimulated, for Olds quickly learned that he could direct the rat to any place in the enclosure simply by pushing the shock button when the animal was at that spot. The rat would haunt the location from then on.

Olds and his colleagues concluded that they had found some sort of "reward" center—they did not use the word pleasure. He then set out to identify other centers of reward by putting his rats through a series of experiments in a Skinner box (named after its inventor, Harvard psychologist B. F. Skinner), which measures the rewarding effect of a stimulus. It consists of a large box, bare except for a pedal that the animal can manipulate; every time the animal pushes the pedal it is rewarded, usually with a pellet of food. How often it pushes the pedal provides an objective measure of the food's value as a reward. For his experiments, Olds held out the promise of an unprecedented kind of reward. He hooked up the pedal to electrodes planted in the rat's brain. The rat's reward for pushing the pedal was electrical stimulation of its own pleasure centers. The results were spectacular.

The rats staged orgies of self-stimulation, their intensity depending on the brain spot stimulated. The most desirable were in the hypothalamus itself. With electrodes accurately planted there, rats pumped the pedal with hardly a pause, some of them up to 5,000 times an hour. They would go on stimulating themselves as many as 2,000 times an hour for 24 consecutive hours, drop from exhaustion, then drag their weary bodies back to the pedal for yet more. Though food and sex were made available, the rats preferred the reward of brain stimulation. They would do almost anything to get at the pedal, even hop across a painfully electrified grid. The insatiable demands of reward centers hint at the grasp of addiction in humans—severe penalties may be ignored when drugs, gambling or other behavior patterns hold promise of attractive reward.

Over the years Olds has mapped what he calls a river of reward running through the hypothalamus. It consists not of discrete centers but of bundled nerve fibers that his electrodes have tapped, much as a telephone trunk line might be tapped at various points between Amsterdam and Paris. Entwined in the same bundle with pleasure appear to be the nerve circuits for many basic drives—the hunger, anger and other feelings that powerfully affect behavior. Their close proximity is not so strange as it might appear at first; the pleasure sites probably serve to reinforce the other drives, making certain an individual is rewarded when he acts to satisfy requirements such as eating, drinking and sex, which ensure the species' survival. Indeed, Olds has found that when his rats are hungry, their appetite for stimulation of the pleasure centers increases. And tampering with a male rat's libido also affects the pleasure centers: castration wipes out the desire for stimulation; injections of the male sex hormone restore it.

Olds' unique behavioral experiments also have confirmed the existence of the punishment sites first located by the Yale group. Rats with electrodes implanted in those sites would push the foot pedal once and respond with classic aversion behavior, assiduously avoiding the foot pedal thereafter. Rats appear to have roughly equal areas of the deep brain devoted to punishment and pleasure. Cats appear to have far more punishment sites—one explanation, perhaps, for the melancholy personalities some people attribute to them. Though stimulation during brain surgery has confirmed that humans also possess centers for both punishment and pleasure, the ratio of the two is still a mystery.

One discovery about feelings in animals should come as no surprise to observers of human nature. In some areas in and around the hypothalamus the distinction between punishment and pleasure seems hopelessly blurred. Stimulation at these points is both pleasant and unpleasant. In one experiment at Yale the rat was given an opportunity to switch on the stimulation by pressing a foot pedal, then switch it off by turning a wheel. It did both, rushing from pedal to wheel and back again, as if uncertain which feeling it preferred—pleasure or pain. James Olds has since suggested that the electrodes were hitting the juncture between the centers of reward and punishment.

Experiments like those that revealed the hypothalamus to be a playground of emotions have also detected centers of strong feelings in its neighboring structures in the limbic system. This entire region near the top of the brain stem is enmeshed in nerve connections, making possible intricately complex byplay between the hypothalamus and other brain structures. These nerves seem to form individual circuits concerned with a particular drive, each circuit employing a specific transmitter substance to carry electric signals across the synaptic gap between its nerve cells *(Chapter 2)*. But the circuits are so closely bundled together that different chemical injections into one site in a male rat's brain can cause him to eat, drink or build nests.

One striking repository of feelings is the amygdala, an almond-shaped component of the limbic system embedded deep in the temporal lobe. When it is stimulated electrically, it can trigger either angry aggression or docility, depending on which part of it is affected.

The amygdala's role in aggression has inspired a number of exper-

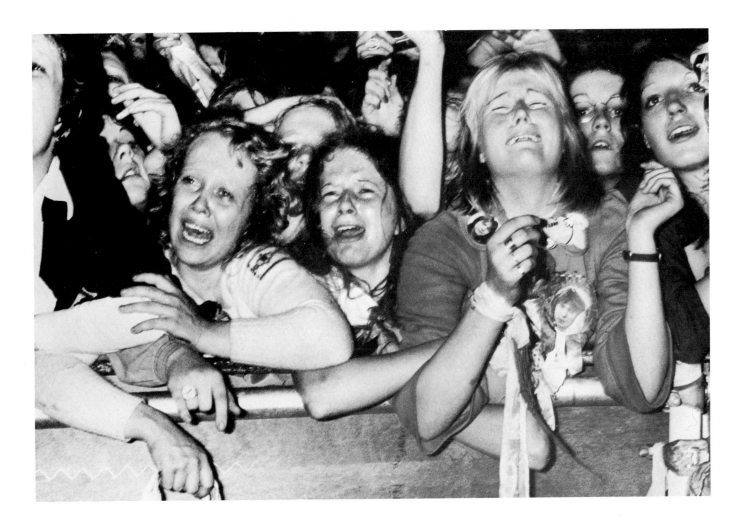

Mob hysteria like that of these teenagers at a London rock concert causes the brain's hypothalamus to order the release of hormones that stimulate the heartbeat. Eventually, the heart may flag and the blood supply to the brain may drop so that fainting results. At this concert 800 people fainted.

iments. When the right spot is touched, a monkey will become calm even in the presence of natural enemies such as the snake. A killer rat will no longer stalk mice. A ferocious bobcat will eat out of the experimenter's hand like a tame tabby.

Even more startling is the outcome of a split-brain experiment on a normally aggressive monkey. Researchers cut the connection between the animal's two cerebral hemispheres and rearranged its optic nerves so that the right eye sent information only to its right brain, the left eye only to the left brain. Then they removed the amygdala from its right temporal lobe. The result was what might almost be called a schizoid monkey. It was normally aggressive when approached on the left side, which reported to the amygdala in the left brain. But it was docile when approached on the right side because the rage-generating amygdala had been removed from the right brain. The amygdala has many connections to the hypothalamus, and the organ's centers of docility and anger apparently influence each other. When a cat was stimulated in the anger center of the hypothalamus, it attacked rats; when it was simultaneously stimulated in the docility center of the amygdala, it stopped the attack. The amygdala's limbic system neighbor, the hippocampus —which affects the process of memory formation (*Chapter 4*)—also can trigger similar feelings when certain of its areas are electrically stimulated. Happily, there is also a cheerful spot in this region of the brain. The thalamus, if stimulated during surgery, can make even the most gravely ill patient smile or laugh out loud.

Along with the precise location of centers of feelings in the brain has come a clearer understanding of the way these centers operate. Much of this detailed knowledge applies to the hypothalamus, perhaps simply because it is the most influential of the brain's emotional structures. This collection of several related groups of nerve cells at the center of the brain is no larger than the tip of the thumb, yet it controls so much of human activity that it has been called a brain within a brain. It governs behavior through three mechanisms: chemical hormone messengers that influence how sluggish, excited or sexy a person feels; the special nervous system that speeds up the heart during stress; and specific centers related to hunger and sex.

The hypothalamus is directly responsible for innate biological drives that are most fundamental to survival—those that keep the body supplied with the warmth and energy essential to life. These nerve cells regulate the behavior of the body's internal environment.

One of these regulators is a thermostat that maintains the body temperature at a constant 98.6° F. winter and summer, in arctic cold and desert heat. The thermostat receives information from two sources. Millions of tiny nerve ends in the skin report on external conditions of heat and cold, and at the same time the bloodstream, washing through the body, reports on the slightest temperature change in the internal organs. Like the thermostat for a combined heating-air conditioning system in a home, the body's thermostat in the hypothalamus compares the two sets of data and orders into action whatever regulatory mechanisms may be needed. If the body is too hot, it triggers activities designed to cool it—sweating and an increase in the flow of blood to the surface of the skin. If the body is cool, it orders shivering and a decreased blood flow. By such means the body's thermostat enables man to survive without clothing in temperatures as low as −20° F. and as high as 100° F.

Rising body temperatures bring into play a second hypothalamic regulator, which controls thirst. Apparently responding principally to the concentration of salt in the bloodstream, this regulator consists of two

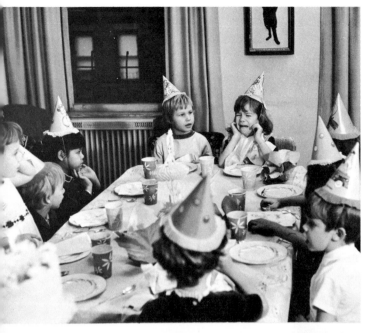
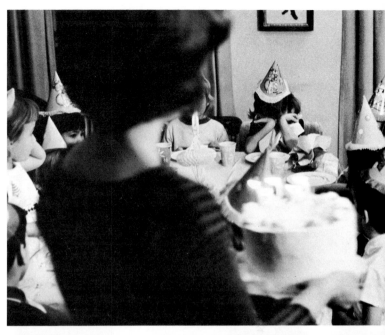
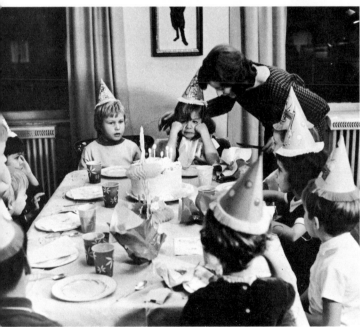
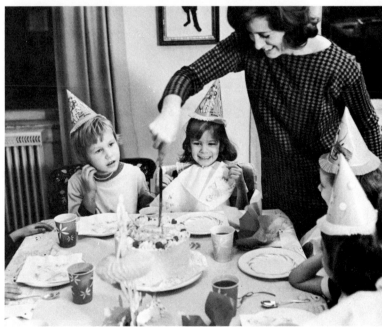

The brain's conscious control over
emotions in young children is so uncertain
that a five-year-old girl gets feelings
mixed up at her birthday party
—inappropriately breaking into tears
(top left and right) when her guests sing
"Happy Birthday." But then she is
consoled (lower left), and smiles as her
mother has trouble cutting the ice cream
cake. As the child grows older, her
emotions will be more controlled.

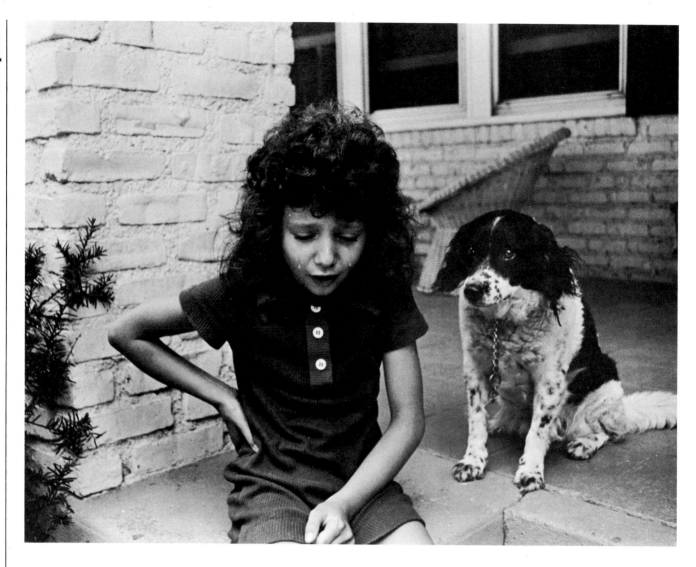

mechanisms—one triggered by high concentrations, the other by low. Injections of salt water in the hypothalamus of an animal make it drink; but if plain water is injected, the animal will temporarily lose interest in drinking even if it has been deprived of water for many hours.

Another pair of regulators in the hypothalamus manages behavior concerned with eating. One, the "appestat," signals hunger and sets off the complex of actions required to get food; the other generates a feeling of satiety to discourage eating. Both apparently arrive at their conclusions not by sensory connections to the stomach, as might be supposed, but by measuring the blood's concentration of glucose, a form of sugar, as it passes through the hypothalamus.

Electrical or chemical stimulation of an animal's appestat hunger center brings on all the symptoms of an empty stomach and sets off the ritual of exploring for food. Destruction of the satiety center removes the built-in limit on eating and makes animals become so obese they scarcely are able to move around small cages. In humans, malfunctions of the hypothalamus can cause such compulsive overeating that one victim even raided the dog biscuit jar.

But being fat or thin ordinarily has little to do with the hypothalamus. For one thing, humans—unlike animals—are not hemmed in by the hypothalamus' demands. Most people can deal with the hunger drive in a couple of ways—by indulging it; or, after a look at a bulging waistline, either by overriding the visceral brain with conscious orders to abstain; or by diverting the brain with thoughts that do not involve food.

The hypothalamus takes direct action only in the most elemental behavior. But indirectly it has a pervasive influence over most emotions and drives—aggression, fear, pleasure—which it exercises through a complex interaction of nerve signals and hormones, the chemical regulators that govern much of human activity. Only because of this interaction can the experimenters' electric probes, stimulating the hypothalamus, turn off the killer instinct in rats, make a cat frightened of mice and keep an animal interminably pressing a pedal for pleasurable signals to its brain.

Hormones, secreted by glands throughout the body, regulate behavior as they chemically govern the deep rhythms of life. The gonads, for instance, produce sex hormones that rule the reproductive cycle; hormones from the thyroid gland in the neck determine whether a person is listless or energetic. Most of the body's glands—each secreting hormones that control specific behavior—take their orders via other hormones from the master gland, the pituitary. One pituitary hormone launches the female reproductive cycle by stimulating the production of estrogen, a hormone that then sets off a chain reaction of hormone production triggering the release of eggs from the ovaries; certain birth-control pills prevent conception by interfering with the mechanism that controls the pituitary's hormone output.

Though the pituitary is anatomically part of the brain—it hangs like a tiny twin-lobed grape from the forward underside of the brain—it was long believed to operate independently. Scientists now have established that the pituitary is the servant of its neighbor in the brain, the hypothalamus. The supervision is carried out by at least two means: the hypothalamus sends electrical impulses through the half-inch long stalk of nerve fibers connecting the two structures and it also releases chemical hormone messages into the blood vessels linking them.

There may also be a third intermediary between pituitary and hypothalamus, ingeniously combining nerve signals and hormones. Nerve cells in the hypothalamus manufacture substances that are much like hormones and can be turned into them. One of these hormone substitutes apparently travels down the axon of the nerve cell, across the synaptic gap and into the pituitary, where it is modified and released into the bloodstream as a hormone. Precisely what *that* hormone does is debatable, but scientists do know that damage to the nerve cells involved with it can result in a type of diabetes marked by the consumption and excretion of vast quantities of water. Another hormone substitute made by nerve cells in the hypothalamus and sent down the nerve fibers is responsible for one of motherhood's many little miracles: if a baby's cries reach his mother's ears, milk leaks from her breasts even when she is sleeping and does not waken.

A remarkable collaboration between hormones and nerves helps govern behavior under stress, when danger, anxiety or a difficult decision demands action. At such moments people say the adrenalin is flowing. The sudden pumping of adrenal hormones prepares the organism for fight or flight, drastic reactions built in by evolution to ensure survival in a hostile world. It speeds up heartbeat, raises blood pressure, relaxes the bronchial tubes to make rapid breathing easier, increases the supply of blood sugar available for energy and triggers the secretion of a long list of other stimulating hormones. It also slows down the digestive process to conserve energy for the muscles (possibly one cause of the anxious feeling of butterflies in the stomach). All these actions are focused on a single purpose: to make available the optimum physical conditions for coping with a state of emergency.

The immediate source of adrenal stress hormones—there are two, norepinephrine and epinephrine—is a gland near the kidney, but the order that sets them flowing originates in the hypothalamus, which receives reports about an impending emergency through its connections with the rest of the brain, including receptors for sight, hearing and smell. The hypothalamus accomplishes more, for it does not rely on the gland alone to protect life in an emergency. At the same time that the hypothalamus signals the adrenal gland to release its fight-or-flight hormones, this brain center also orders into action a parallel set of preparations for emergency action. It generates signals that go directly to many parts of the body, duplicating the orders of the hormones to change heart rate and muscle tension. The nerve signals also take some protective steps the hormones do not, such as alerting the eyes and the ears to watch and listen more closely. This parallel control, employing two systems to handle one kind of behavior, is unique; it may have evolved because stress actions are so essential to survival. The intimate rela-

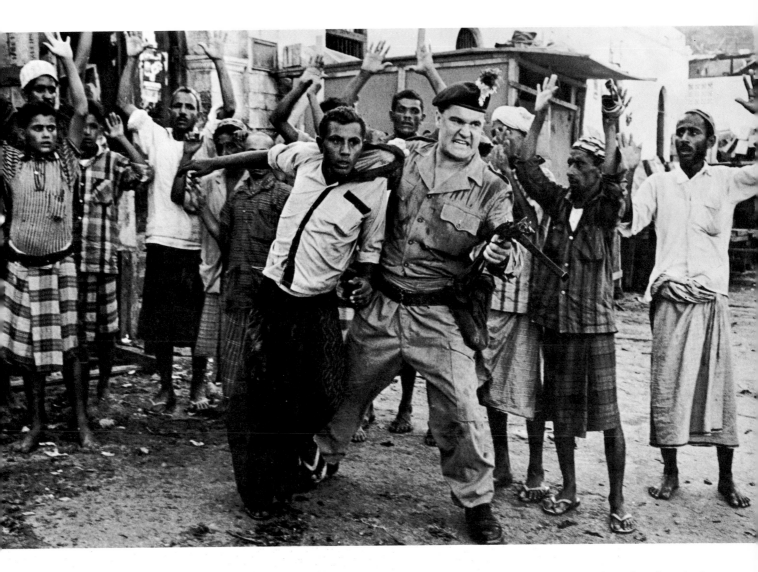

Anger and fear appear together following the explosion of a terrorist's grenade in strife-torn Aden—an enraged British soldier, gun in hand, restrains one demonstrator while onlookers stand back in fear and submission. The two emotions are related—they are modulated by neighboring structures in the limbic system (page 110).

tionship between the two systems is clearly reflected in the chemicals they use: stress nerve signals are transmitted from nerve cell to nerve cell by the neurotransmitter norepinephrine—exactly the same substance released by the adrenal gland.

The interaction between hormones and the brain is much more subtle in sexual behavior. The hypothalamus controls the release of sex hormones, as it does adrenal hormones, but the sex hormones in turn help control the actions of the hypothalamus. The hormones only help, however, for sensory nerve signals also stimulate the hypothalamus and cause more hormones to be released. This intertwined pattern of circular processes is common knowledge, of course—the sight of a pretty girl sets any young man's heart beating faster.

But the pattern is also amply confirmed in laboratory tests of animals. Experiments demonstrate that the simple act of seeing the

121

opposite sex can bring instantaneous changes in the level of sex hormones. A message noting that a desirable creature has arrived on the scene is flashed to the hypothalamus via the optic nerve. The hypothalamus promptly directs release of hormones that tell the heart muscles to speed up. The sequence will continue to develop as the external situation dictates, eventually bringing into play all the behavior of courtship, mating, nest building and parental care.

The sex hormone's influence on feelings extends beyond sexual behavior. In women the hormone levels rise and fall in a regular sequence, following the monthly cycle dictated by the built-in calendar in the circuits of the hypothalamus. This cycle causes changes in feeling and need. Most people are aware of the irritability and depression in women that often mark the two or three days before the onset of menstruation. Experiments also show that at this time the substance of a woman's dreams may be unusually aggressive and sensual. One study conducted among women convicts indicates that a female's likelihood of committing a crime appears to be four times greater than normal in the days just preceding menstruation.

The most extraordinary effect of sex hormones upon drives and emotions is gender itself—the feeling that makes men behave like men, and women like women. A man's brain is not precisely the same as a woman's. And yet they both started out alike. When conception starts the embryo brain developing, it begins female—regardless of whether the baby is to be a boy or a girl. The brain apparently becomes male only if a certain male sex hormone acts upon it at a critical stage in development. In rats this period occurs in the first four days after birth. In monkeys —and presumably humans—it occurs before birth, while the embryo is still in the womb.

The experiments that first brought this information to light in 1965 tell much about the development of behavior. They involved baby rats that were physically male. During the first four days after birth their sex glands were removed, depriving them of the male sex hormone testosterone. Though the sexual organs themselves remained unchanged, the young male rats developed a female cycle of hormone production precisely as if they were to ovulate and menstruate. Their behavior also tended to coincide with patterns associated with the female reproductive cycle. One barometer of this is the amount of running a rat will do on an activity wheel. Normal males are uniformly active from day to day. Female activity follows a cycle, peaking at the time of ovulation. So did that of the experimental males. Moreover, when the males were later given small doses of female sex hormones, they displayed the sexual activities of females. The gender-changing effects of the male sex hormone were confirmed in female rats. Unlike male rats, who were deprived of testosterone, the females were given doses of it, and grew up to behave like males, acting out the entire male sex ritual.

These remarkable findings may have enormous implications for the study of human sexual behavior. So-called transsexuals—people who develop gender feelings at odds with their physical sex, apparently because of a genetic abnormality—can be treated with surgery and hormones to bring physique and feelings into accord. Hormonal imbalances seem to be involved in some cases of homosexuality. And it is true that injections of male hormones often strengthen waning sexual feelings in old men.

The mapping of centers of emotion and the analysis of their operation have opened a whole new frontier in the study of the brain and behavior. Manipulation of these areas—electrically, chemically and surgically—is now a principal instrument for examining and shaping animal behavior in the laboratory, and it is being used on humans as well. Predictably, the latter approach has raised grave moral questions.

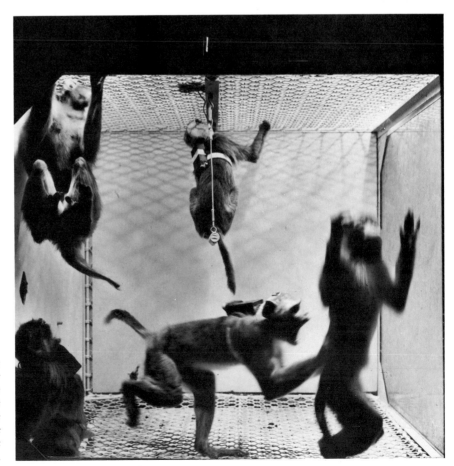

Electrical stimulation of the brain causes this monkey to fly into a rage and scatter his companions in a cage during a Yale experiment that located circuits controlling aggression. Electrodes were implanted in the monkey's thalamic region and activated by radio signals sent to a receiver on the animal's back.

One of the leaders in animal experimentation—and a foremost exponent of manipulation of human emotions—is José Delgado, a member of the Yale team that found the punishment centers in the brain. Widely known for the flamboyance of his experiments, Delgado staged a particularly dramatic demonstration in Cordova in his native Spain in 1964. He stood alone in a bull ring and stopped a bull in mid-charge by pressing a button on a radio control to turn on electrodes implanted in the bull's brain. With similar stimulation of the deep brain, Delgado has made one monkey go through the paces of an intricate behavioral sequence 20,000 times in a row; he has made another one smile 400,000 times; and he has taught the mate of a tyrannical monkey named Ali to pacify him by pushing a button, triggering electrical stimulation in his amygdala rage center.

Delgado has devised an entire arsenal of gadgetry for the electrical and chemical manipulation of behavior. One device, which he calls a dialytrode, permits mind-affecting chemicals to be stored in silicone rubber bags under the scalp, then delivered a drop at a time to behavioral centers. But his best-known invention is a radio transmitter and receiver called the stimoceiver. No bigger than a postage stamp, the stimoceiver was connected to electrodes in the brain and permanently anchored on the top of the skull of a chimp named Paddy. It monitored the brain's electrical activity and transmitted the information to a computer 300 feet away. The computer analyzed the signals, and if it detected brain waves thought to be associated with aggressiveness, the computer signaled the stimoceiver to punish Paddy. The stimoceiver automatically switched on electrodes in the punishment centers around the hypothalamus. After a couple of unpleasant jolts, Paddy learned to remain so placid that his aggressive instincts were not even aroused by threats from other chimps.

These methods, Delgado maintains in his book, *Physical Control of the Mind*, should be used on human brains to create a happier, less destructive and "psychocivilized society." To illustrate the power of such techniques, Delgado describes an experience with electrodes inserted in the motor control centers of a patient suffering from epilepsy. The electrodes forced the man to make a fist, though he kept trying to extend his fingers. Delgado quotes the patient as saying, "I guess, Doctor, that your electricity is stronger than my will."

Such attempts to intervene in the brain's control over behavior do not depend on space-age gadgets like Delgado's radio-operated electrodes. History is full of attempts—mostly disastrous—to manipulate human feelings with surgery, drugs and a variety of other methods. In earlier

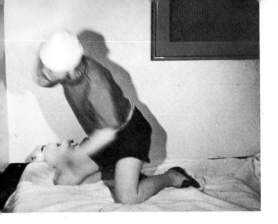

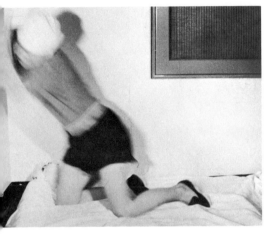

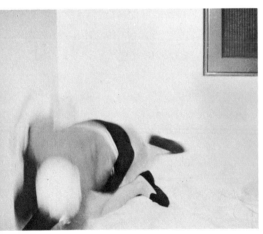

To localize the source of trouble in a brain-damaged patient who repeatedly became violent, Boston physicians implanted electrodes in several areas of her brain. When they stimulated one area —the amygdala—the girl rose to her knees (top), pounded the wall in a frenzy (middle), then slumped down again (bottom). Surgeons later removed brain tissue in the area and the patient began to lead a more normal life.

times, emotional control took the form of castration (effective because it eliminates the source of male sex hormones) and even removal of the large intestine (ineffective). In 1891 a Swiss surgeon, Gottlieb Burckhardt, reported that he could eliminate "exciting impulses" by cutting out brain portions of mental patients, but he soon abandoned that approach after criticism from his colleagues. His idea was picked up again in the 1930s in the form of frontal lobotomy, an operation for the removal of part of the front of the brain to calm violent mental patients and relieve their hallucinations.

The chief proponent of lobotomies was a Portuguese diplomat and psychiatrist named Egas Moniz, who heard a report on research at Yale in which pieces of the front brain had been removed from two chimpanzees, Becky and Lucy. The surgery had rendered the once quarrelsome pair into very placid chimps; in the words of the report: "The apes acted as though they had joined the happiness cult . . . and placed their burdens on the Lord."

The taming of Becky and Lucy convinced Moniz that front-brain surgery could relieve his psychotic human patients of their delusions and hallucinations—in spite of the fact that there was very little evidence to back his belief.

Little is known for certain about the front brain, although it appears to be involved in planning and foresight. For nearly a century one of the few clues that it might affect personality was the celebrated example of Phineas Gage. A 19th Century railroad worker whose skull is still on display at Harvard, Gage had an inch-thick iron rod blasted through his head. Though much of his front brain was destroyed, Gage miraculously survived with memory and thought intact. People who knew him, however, said he was a changed man—"no longer Gage." Once mild-spoken, steady and efficient, he became foul-mouthed and fitful, forever changing his plans. His doctor, at a loss for a medical explanation of the change in Gage's personality, said that the hole in the brain had caused an imbalance "between his intellectual faculties and animal propensities."

The disastrous example of Phineas Gage notwithstanding, Moniz persuaded a surgeon colleague to perform a lobotomy on a patient, gouging out with several twists of the scalpel the nerve fibers connecting the frontal lobes to the rest of the brain. The violently psychotic patient did indeed become calm and tractable, and frontal lobotomies were soon being performed in many countries. An estimated 50 per cent were deemed successful; they apparently worked because connections to the deep emotional centers were severed.

But in some instances the operation also brought unattractive side results, destroying the patient's ambition, creativity and sense of responsibility, or even leaving him incapable of any thought. Not all subjects were hopeless mental patients. A lawyer who was anxious about his bouts of violent drinking submitted to a lobotomy. The surgery removed his anxieties about drinking but did not stop him from getting violently drunk.

By the 1950s lobotomies were largely supplanted by the safer and more effective tranquilizing drugs, but surgery to control emotional behavior continued. It has become more precise and knowledgeable, but it generates even more controversy than ever. In Germany, surgeons have destroyed the sex centers of the hypothalamus as a court-sanctioned alternative to imprisonment for sexual deviants. In Japan, bits of either the hypothalamus or the amygdala have been eliminated with electric needles to control assaultive behavior in a large number of children and adults, and the same technique has been used several times for similar cases in the United States.

One American patient, Julia, a musically talented young woman, had spent most of her life in prisons and mental hospitals. She had attacked 10 persons, nearly killed two others and tried suicide four times. Before surgeons burned out an area of her amygdala, they implanted electrodes there to study her behavior. A quick burst of current so enraged her that she smashed her guitar against the hospital wall, barely missing the psychiatrist's head. Surgery had a calming effect and enabled her to live at home instead of in an institution. The results in other cases have been mixed: some patients have remained free of violence; others have suffered further attacks of rage.

More provocative than surgical removal of brain tissue is a practice that until recently seemed the province of science fiction: permanently implanting electrodes in the emotional centers of human beings. Robert Heath of Tulane University inserted electrodes in the brain of mental patients to provide pleasure, a feeling Heath believed they were deprived of by a defect in the area near the hypothalamus. Some patients carried their own battery power sources and control boxes, and were free to stimulate themselves. The result of this stimulation, the patients reported, ranged from mild euphoria to what was described as "better than sex." But the stimulation also seemed to elicit an odd compulsiveness. In several instances, patients went on pushing the button after the electricity had been turned off.

Such tampering with the brain worries many scientists not only because it might threaten basic human freedoms, but also because they question its practical value. They feel understanding of the deep brain is still fragmentary, the evidence from animal experiments often ambiguous and contradictory. The circuits of emotion are so closely intertwined that stimulation or surgery is likely to overlap several circuits and bring undesirable results. The effects of electrical stimulation, like those of drugs, may depend upon mood, personality and even the practitioner's own enthusiasm.

Most of all, many scientists believe it is impossible to tamper with one slice of behavior without doing damage to the entire pie. One bizarre case illustrates the dangers. According to a well-publicized account, an engineer who reputedly became the model for the electronically manipulated protagonist of the novel *The Terminal Man* suffered terrible outbursts of violence. He would accuse his wife of "carrying on" with a neighbor and hurl her against the wall. Once he burned her chest with a cigarette.

He sought treatment, and 22 electrodes were implanted in his brain to locate the source of his irrational rage. When an electrode in one portion of his amygdala was switched on, the patient announced: "I am losing control." When a second electrode, about one sixth of an inch away, was turned on, he described a druglike euphoria: "I'm feeling in a good mood now . . . a feeling like Demerol . . . like I am floating on a cloud." The euphoric spot was stimulated every day for three months and the patient stayed free of his uncontrollable rage. Finally, with his consent, the anger spot was burned out.

But a follow-up study of the case provided a tragic sequel. His wife filed for divorce and eventually married their neighbor—the one whom the patient, in his previous bouts of rage, had accused her of "carrying on" with. Soon after, he was confined to a hospital for psychiatric reasons. One of the symptoms of his disturbed state was his belief that electrodes had been placed in his brain so that, the hospital record states, "they can control him, control his moods and control his actions, they can turn him up or turn him down."

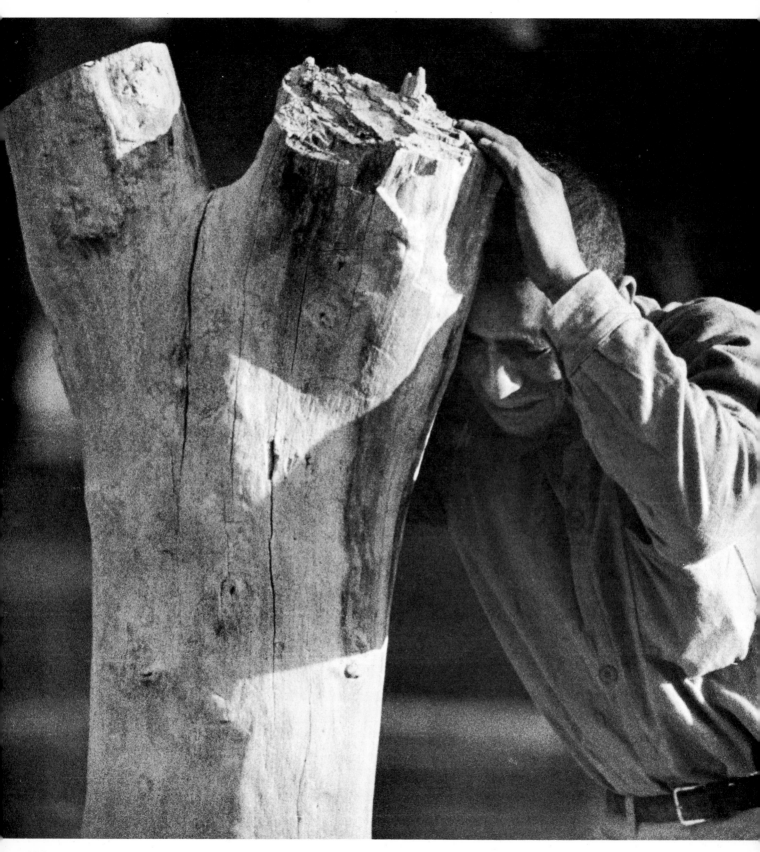

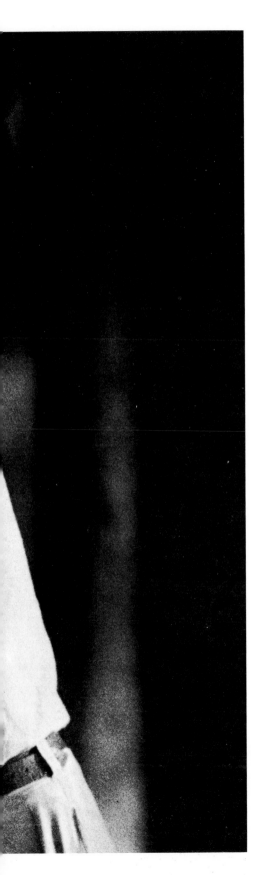

Coping with emotions

Three basic emotions—anger, fear and pleasure—are largely the province of the limbic system, a thick, doughnut-shaped mass of nerve cells encircling the top of the brain stem. These emotions evolved as aids to self-preservation and they still serve that function. A feeling of anger increases the alertness, endurance and strength of a man who finds himself in a situation where he has to fight for his life; fear, on the other hand, can arouse him to run from danger before it is too late. Pleasure or the promise of pleasure leads him to seek out the food that will sustain his body and the sexual activity that will perpetuate his species.

But intense emotions—and the racing heart, sweating palms and knotted stomach that go with them—can sometimes be both inconvenient and uncomfortable. An individual often tries to deal with them by denying them, and he may unconsciously suppress his feelings before he becomes aware that they have been aroused.

Though a deliberate control of the emotions is often unavoidable, unconscious suppression can be dangerous. So powerful are the basic emotions that they may simply erupt in other more painful forms, causing psychological conflicts or else psychosomatic illnesses from ulcers to asthma. Generally healthier are the types of emotional release shown on these and the following pages, in which men, women and children in the grip of strong emotions give vent to their feelings in overt behavior. Allowing feelings to be expressed openly helps to restore the individual to a state of equilibrium, draining off the tension that emotions such as anger, anxiety and even ecstasy can produce.

Wracked by a paroxysm of grief, a Turkish villager on the island of Cyprus sobs uncontrollably on returning to his home after a 1963 night raid by Greek forces and finding that his entire family has been killed.

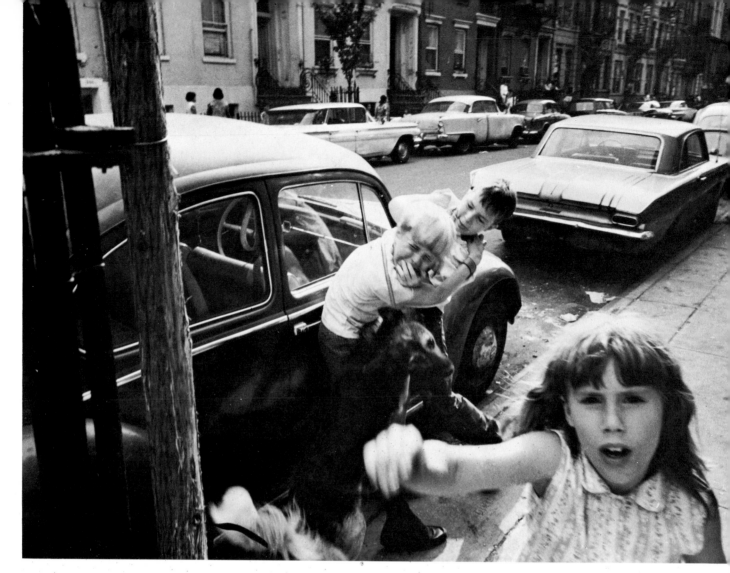

An explosion of aggression

The classic method of releasing anger is a frenzied physical attack upon the object, animate or inanimate, that has aroused that emotion. Sigmund Freud believed that this resort to direct aggression was the oldest of all expressions of anger. Certainly it is the first way of expressing anger to be learned by human beings: children begin to display uncontrolled aggression when they reach the age of two.

Why use aggression to release anger? The German animal behaviorist Konrad Lorenz has theorized that human aggression is an instinctive drive surviving from prehistoric times, when it helped man to obtain food and to defend his home territory. Lorenz's theories, like Freud's, are controversial, but the sequence of pictures on these pages shows that territorial encroachment can still start a fight—though the ground to be defended is a city block rather than an age-old African plain.

A no-holds-barred battle between two boys breaks out when the blond boy, who has walked his dog onto the block where the dark-haired boy lives, defies the latter's order to move on. As the tussle grows more desperate, the sister of the dark-haired boy runs for help.

As the battle moves out into the street, the furious invader attacks with an improvised club, and the territorial defender uses an equally improvised shield against his enemy and the dog. In the end, block residents broke up the scrap and sent the trespasser safely home.

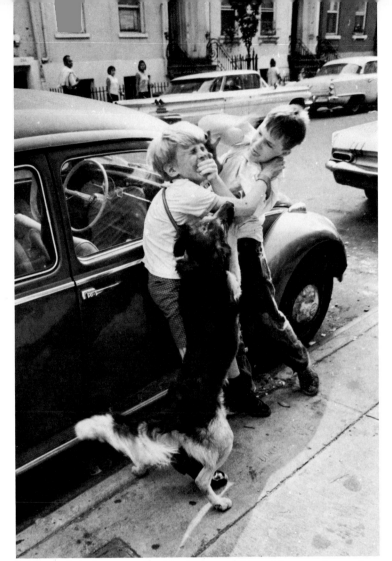

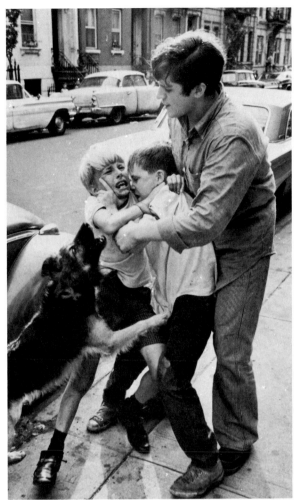

The intruder's dog enters into the fray, snapping at his master's attacker.

An adult passerby cannot separate the two combatants.

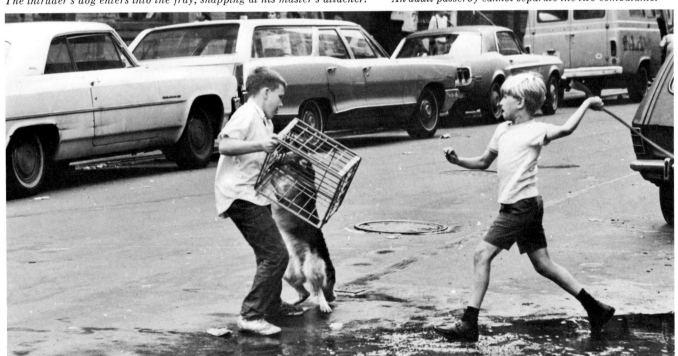

Thrills and relief in fun and games

Recreation, particularly games and organized sports, serves as an outlet for emotions everywhere. Violent exercise seems to act as a natural tranquilizer, and acute anxiety before a game gives way to an exhilarating sense of relief once it starts.

Similarly, the spectator at an event involving violent contact and intense competition may release violent feelings by transferring them to the players, and indulge in mild forms of violence himself. Within the crowd at a stadium he can generally boo and hoot, cheer and stamp until he has rid himself of emotion and regained his inner balance.

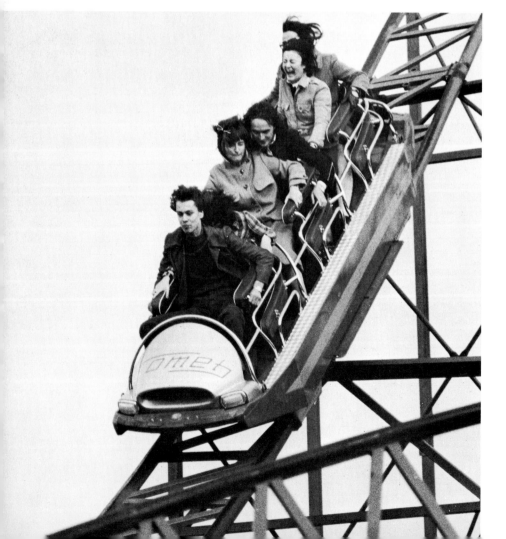

Passengers on a roller coaster in a Viennese amusement park freeze in fear or give way in shrieks as their car plummets down the track. The twists and drops of the roller coaster are deliberately designed to provoke fear without introducing real danger, then to relieve the emotion in a safe return.

In a frenzied dance of joy, a fan at the 1963 All-Ireland Football Final in Dublin expresses and releases ecstasy aroused by the home team's last-minute, one-point victory over Galway. His abandon might not ordinarily be tolerated in public, but it is acceptable and even encouraged among spectators at a sports event.

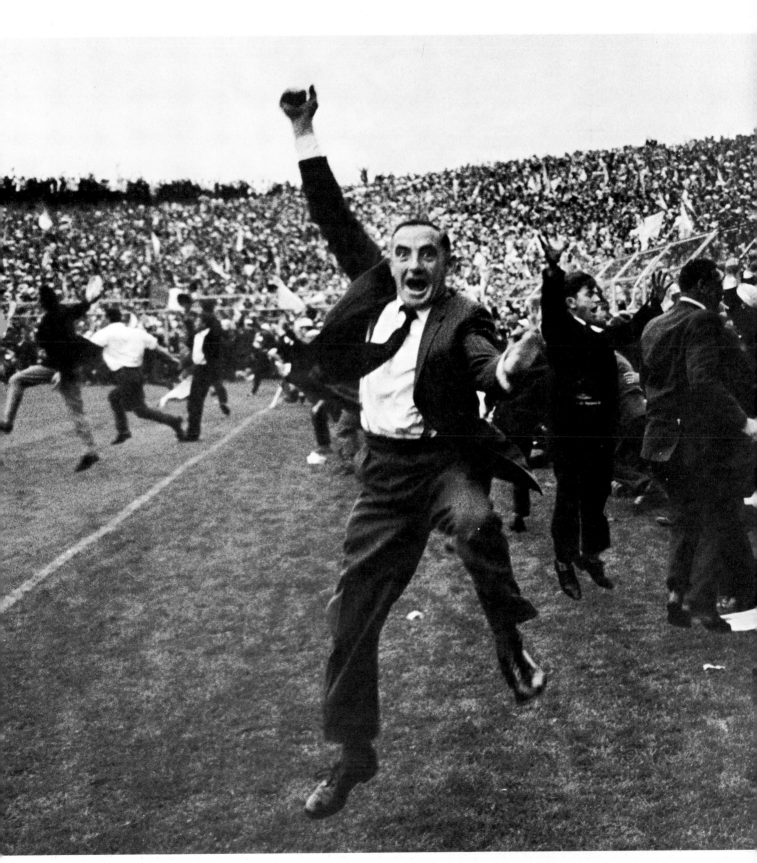

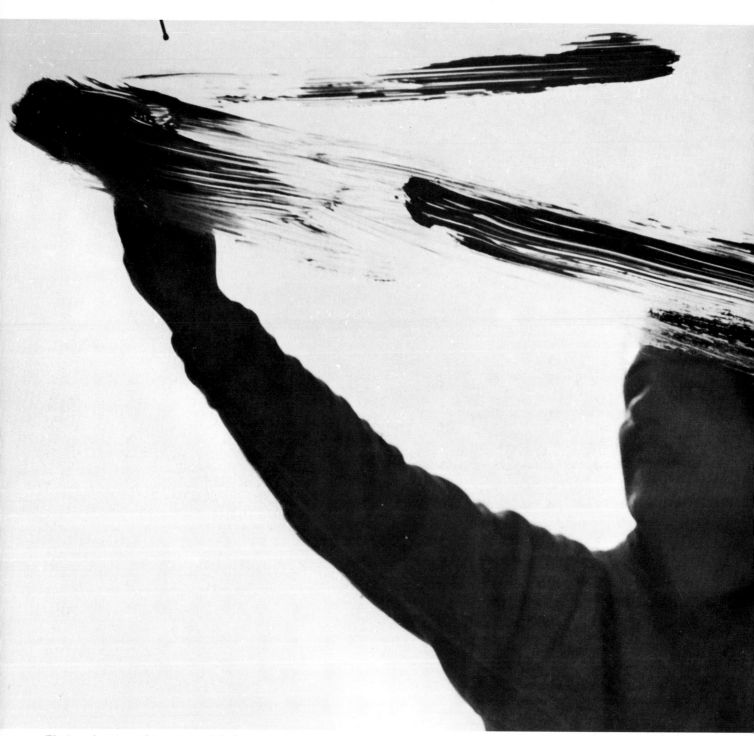

The late American abstract expressionist
Franz Kline transfers his energetic
feelings into explosively sweeping thick
strokes of paint across a sheet of glass.
Kline once said: "The final test of a
painting, theirs, mine, any other, is: does
the painter's emotion come across?"

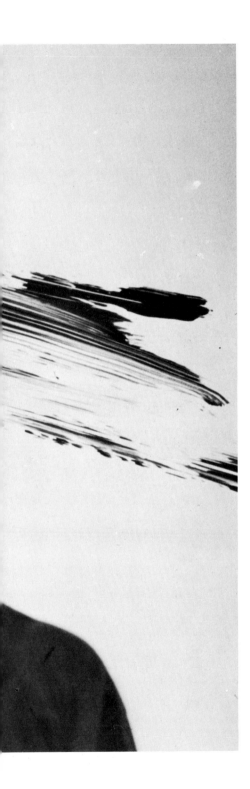

An outlet in creativity

Artists have a most effective method of handling emotion: they convert it into art. A good example is the actor, who uses his own emotions to project those of the character he plays.

The 19th Century English poet William Wordsworth spoke for all writers when he defined poetry as "the spontaneous overflow of powerful feelings" with its origins in "emotion recollected in tranquillity." And the Netherlander Vincent van Gogh, writing of the painter's creative life, asked: "Is it not emotion, the sincerity of one's feeling for nature, that drives us?"

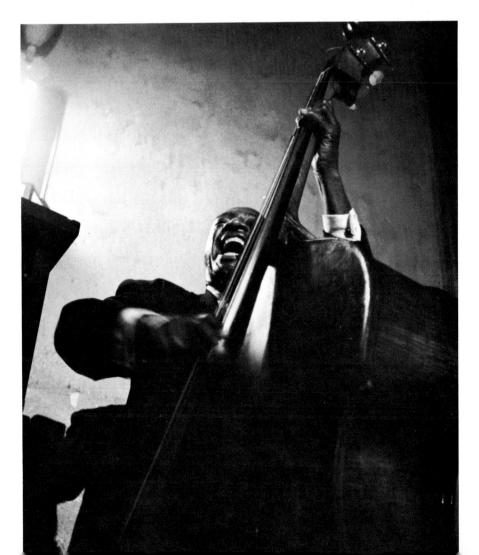

Jazz bassist Milt Hinton contorts his features and closes his eyes during a solo. He explains: "I shut my eyes to concentrate on what I feel. That way I keep the distractions out while I weave what is inside me into song."

Keeping a stiff upper lip

In certain circumstances a conscious and deliberate control over the expression of an emotion may be the most realistic way of dealing with it. A national cult of the stiff upper lip helped the British people endure the German bombings of World War II. When sirens sounded, Londoners walked, not ran, to air-raid shelters—and when they got there, lined up quietly in long queues, serenaded by plucky street singers, as they waited to enter. Equally firm control can protect soldiers from danger (*opposite*) or prepare student nurses for chilling sights (*bottom*).

Members of England's Royal Artillery Display Team react in accordance with the danger as a cyclist hurdles over them. Those at the beginning of the jump smile in noticeable relief, while those at the far end keep a properly stiff upper lip.

Student nurses at their first autopsy stifle repulsion and nausea as a physician-instructor saws open the chest cavity of a cadaver. No one fainted—though some of the students turned a little green.

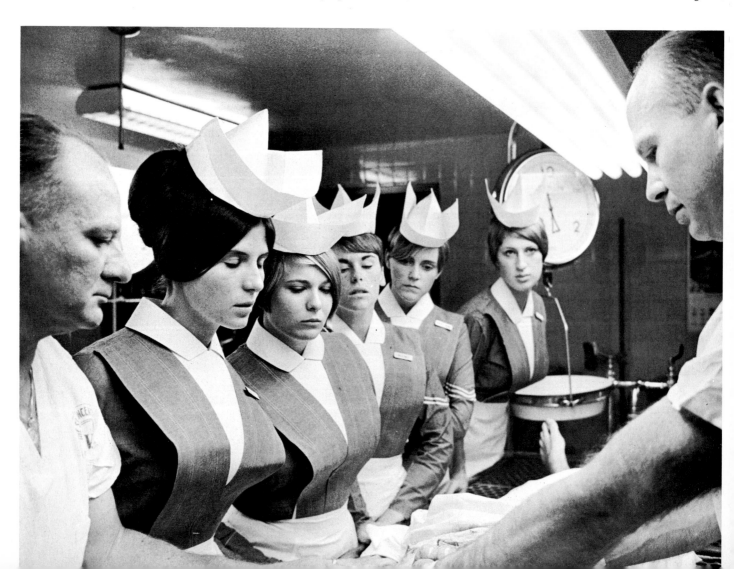

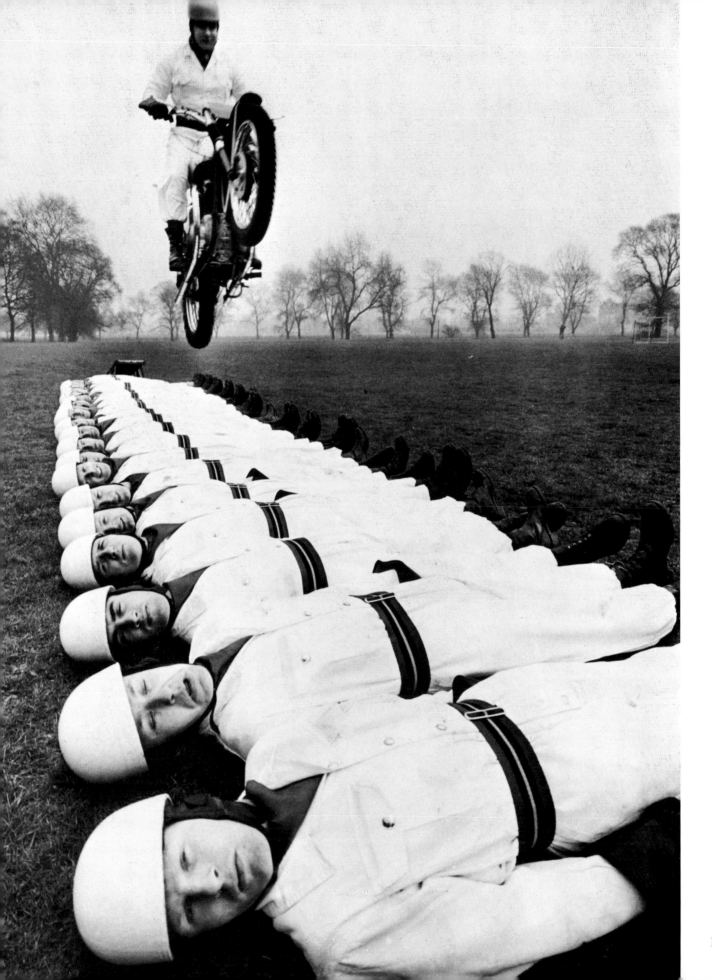

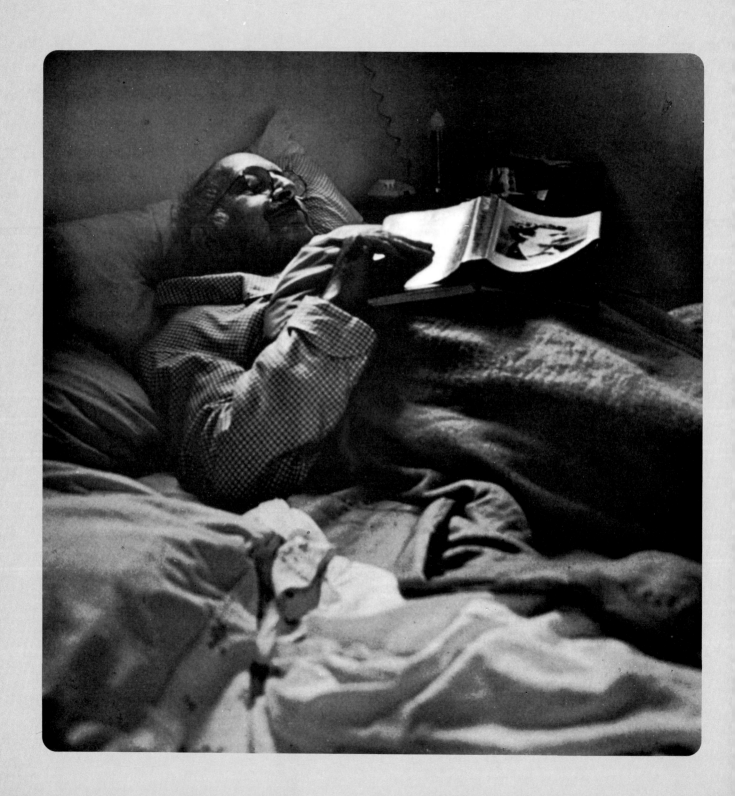

To Sleep, to Dream

The ultimate mystery of the brain, its power to control mental alertness, is finally being solved with clues from a grab bag of sources: the student who noticed that babies' eyes twitch as they slept; the disc jockey who, as a stunt, kept himself awake for 200 hours; the Oriental mystics who exercise mental control over heartbeat and blood pressure. Bits of evidence obtained from these seemingly unrelated sources now fit together to show how the brain shifts from one level of consciousness to another, following the ebb and flow of electrical activity within its 10 billion nerve cells.

The most familiar state of consciousness is the one that dominates the waking hours of most people; it can be characterized as one of alertness and concentration. More rare is the relaxed state of awareness associated with meditation or daydreaming, or simply with those moments when the eyes close and the mind idles. During sleep, once considered a period of total quiescence, the brain fluctuates between two states of awareness, one peaceful and deep, the other turbulent and episodic, akin to wakefulness. It is during this latter state that men dream.

In addition to these four naturally occurring states of awareness, the brain can also be coaxed or catapulted into other states. Man has altered his perception of reality by such means as fasting, hypnotism and religious ritual. He has used drugs like alcohol to induce a state of euphoria, drugs like heroin to lull himself into oblivion, and drugs such as marijuana and LSD to launch himself into hallucinatory states full of bizarre images resembling those of madness. All these states of consciousness, normal and abnormal, affect electrical activity in the brain, as measured by a device called the electroencephalograph, or EEG. When it is connected to wires pasted to the scalp, it records internal changes in voltage, or electrical pressure, graphing these changes on a moving strip of paper as a "brain wave." The patterns of deliberately altered states of consciousness often provide conflicting data, but the graph immediately identifies the four normal consciousness levels: moderate changes of eight to 13 times per second of "alpha waves" for relaxed awareness; more rapid changes of 14 to 30 times per second of the "beta waves" for full alertness; slow waves alternating only one half to three and a half times per second during deep sleep; and a somewhat faster, beta-like frequency during periods of dreaming.

Of these categories of consciousness the two most conspicuous are of course sleep and wakefulness, which follow the 24-hour rhythm of the earth's day. These 24-hour cycles are called circadian rhythms—from the Latin for "about one day." The circadian rhythms remain relatively constant despite changes in external conditions, a fact that is obvious to anyone who travels across time zones in an airliner: the familiar phenomenon of "jet lag" is nothing more than the circadian rhythm's natural inclination to go its own way regardless of what the local clock says. At the same time, within these daily rhythms there are shorter cycles; every 90 minutes or so the brain's attentiveness wanes. During wakefulness, these are the moments when an individual wanders off to the water cooler or craves a sandwich; at night, they are the times that seem to coincide with the most vivid dreams.

To regulate these various rhythms the body needs its own clock. Animal experiments indicate it is the pineal gland, a small object shaped like a pine cone and attached to the top of the brain stem. Early anatomists could only speculate on the function of the pineal—one considered it a valve regulating the flow of thought, another "the seat of the soul." The clue to the pineal's timekeeping function came from the biological role it plays in the behavior of fish and amphibians, where it acts as a light-sensitive third eye. Located at the back of the head just beneath the creature's skin, this third eye registers a dimming in illumination when night falls, triggering the pineal to release hormones that darken and camouflage the creature's skin. In humans as well, the pineal receives information about light and dark, synchronizing it to the day-night cycle outside, but the synchronizing cues arrive by a more circuitous route, through nerve impulses transmitted by the eyes.

As a regulatory device, the pineal has many functions; it triggers puberty in both boys and girls, for instance, and apparently helps to pace the menstrual periods. In the circadian cycle it may order the passage from wakefulness to sleep, for one of the chemicals associated with sleep, serotonin, builds up and subsides markedly in the pineal.

Though the pineal takes its initial cues from the sequence of day and night, its mechanisms, once set, seem to keep fairly correct time without external prompting. Volunteers who have lived in caves and mines without the usual reference to light and dark nevertheless manage to maintain their regular 24-hour cycle of waking and sleeping. The only noticeable difference is a tendency for their biological clocks to run a little slow, so that they occasionally imagine they have been living in the dark for shorter periods of time than is actually the case. Similarly, animals that are raised in the artificial environment of a windowless laboratory follow the circadian rhythms of their species—even though they have never been exposed to the regulatory cues of night and day. Indeed, the giant sea slug *aplysia* follows the 12-hour sleep rhythms of its tidal existence even when it lives in a laboratory tank.

The pineal clock that establishes these day-night rhythms does not abruptly switch the brain from one activity or level of consciousness to another, but rather informs it that the appropriate moment for switching is at hand. The brain then makes up its mind. It may ignore bedtime, and stay awake long past the sleep hour fixed by habit and the earth's revolutions; with a bit more difficulty, it awakens at a time chosen consciously rather than by any secretions of the pineal gland. The actual change in consciousness is accomplished in a different part of the brain, by a network of nerve cells rooted in one small part of the brain stem. This master switch of awareness, no bigger than the little finger, is the reticular activating system, or RAS. It alerts the brain to incoming information from the senses, and from the centers of thought, memory and feeling. More than that, it adjudicates the relative importance of that information permitting the mind to focus on a single stimulus. When a child searches for a four-leaf clover in a sea of grass, the RAS focuses his mind on the object of the search. When an adult wants to read a book in a room full of children, the RAS filters out the din, yet allows him to hear his name spoken from across the room.

In a way the RAS is like a vigilant secretary, sorting out the trivia from the incoming messages. Like a good secretary, it does not block any messages completely; rather, it seems to put a priority tag on some items. As the nerve fibers carrying information to the executive· decision levels at the brain's cortex pass through the RAS, the nerve cells within the RAS fire off their own messages, timing them to arrive simultaneously with the incoming message. Each of these matching messages seems to be carried by an RAS nerve circuit devoted solely to one kind of input. Thus, incoming hearing messages trigger one kind of RAS neuron, while touch messages trigger another.

Clearly, the primary purpose of the RAS is self-preservation, for its unfailing trigger is danger or the threat of danger. Signals, for instance, from such internal functions as breathing and heartbeat pepper the brain

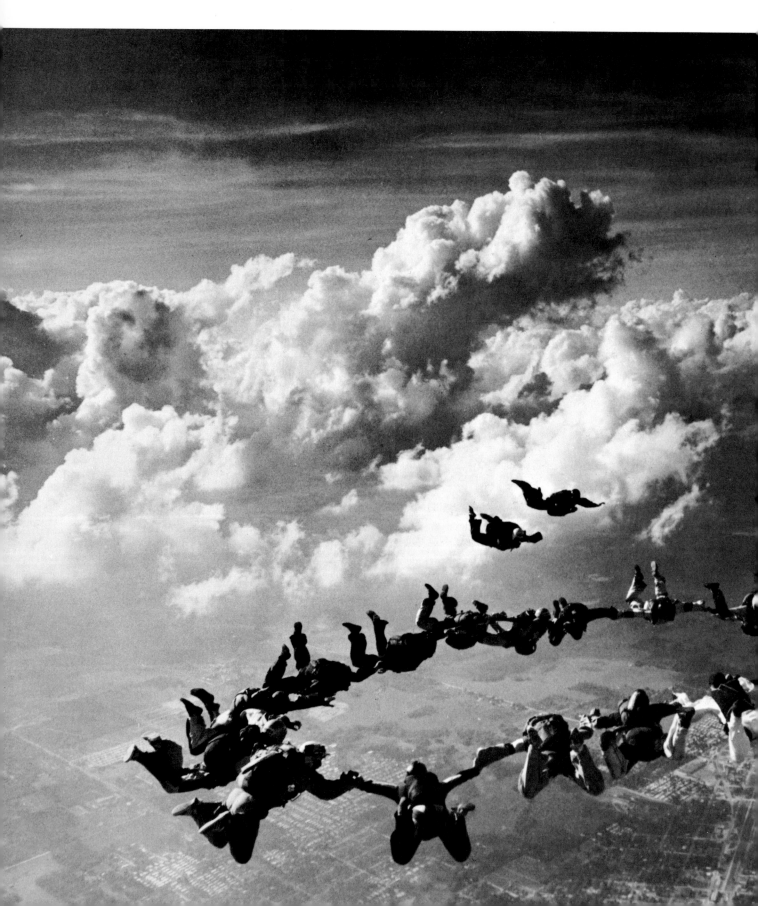

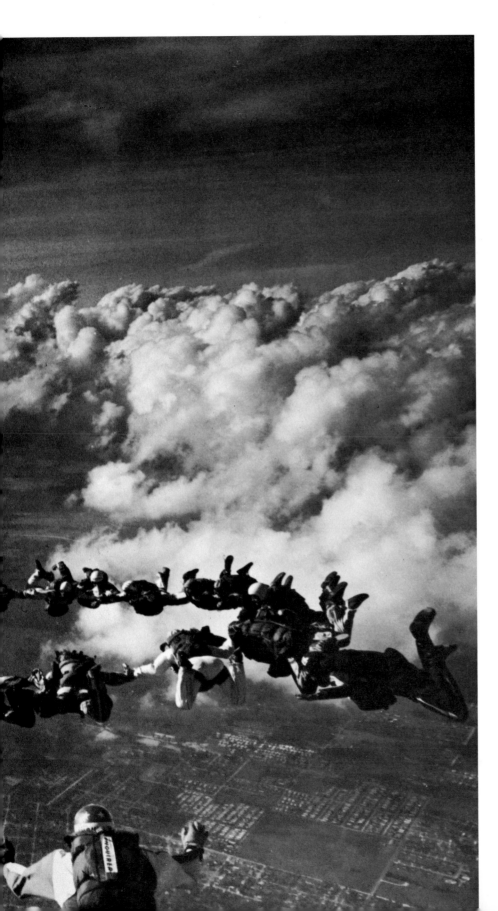

A natural "high" is achieved by a ring of skydivers during a free fall over Florida. The exhilaration of the jump, acting on the brain's reticular activating system, serves as a stimulus to raise their awareness to a euphoria that has been likened to a drug-induced high. A few divers seem to have become so euphoric that they have failed to pull the rip cord —and have fallen to their deaths.

cortex constantly, yet the brain pays little attention to them unless the RAS alerts it that something is wrong. Similarly, a mother will sleep through heavy traffic noise but waken at the faintest cry from her baby, while a sleeping father may not hear a child crying but is likely to be immediately aroused by a whiff of smoke.

Danger is not the only signal that activates the RAS. The smell of food, the sound of music, the sight of a pretty woman—anything that interests the mind turns the switch for alertness. The brain itself stimulates the RAS by thinking—who has not lain wide awake late into the night, alert and anxious and powerless to switch off his RAS? Artificial stimulation also activates the RAS. Psychologists working with monkeys in laboratories have increased alertness, encouraging the animals to learn faster, by stimulating the RAS with electric probes. The so-called learning drugs, such as amphetamine, do much the same thing—by chemical means. And truck drivers, students and night workers who use pep pills to stay awake are also activating the RAS chemically.

It almost seems that the brain craves the kind of sensory excitement that keeps it in the alert beta rhythm. One measure of this thirst is man's insatiable appetite for adventure—for climbing mountains, racing motorcycles, or just watching the action of a football game. Stronger evidence of the RAS's need for activity is the harm that results when it is lacking. If a man is totally deprived of such stimulation, he may become seriously disoriented. In one classic demonstration, a group of student volunteers at McGill University in Montreal were paid to lie in bed and do nothing. They were blindfolded, their ears were covered with ear muffs and their hands were padded with heavy gloves, cutting them off from all sensory stimulation. This dissociation from the world so disturbed several of the volunteers that they quit at the end of the first day, and those who endured to the end of the experiment suffered from hallucinations. One volunteer claimed he heard a church choir singing; another reported seeing a procession of marching squirrels. And any sort of sensory experience, even a painful one, seems better than none at all—young rats that were given a mild shock every day fared much better than those raised without ever being touched.

Continuous excitement, of course, may be as unnerving as a lack of stimulation. The RAS apparently cannot be locked in any of its settings for a prolonged period of time; it normally switches back and forth at regular intervals between the daydreaming alpha rhythm and the alert beta rhythm, and at least twice a day it switches between sleep and wakefulness. Once it was thought that sleep was produced simply by switching off the RAS—but then it was discovered that damage to the RAS caused

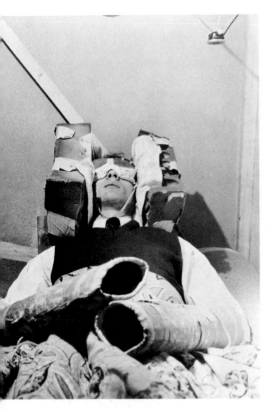

His hearing blocked by ear muffs, his eyes masked to reduce vision, his gloved hands swathed in cardboard cuffs so that he touches nothing, a volunteer in an experiment at McGill University waits to see what will happen when he is deprived of all outside sensory contact. Within a week, most subjects began hallucinating.

complete loss of consciousness. Instead of putting the individual to sleep, it put him into a coma. Thereafter it was found that a second mechanism modulated the RAS, in effect bringing sleep by putting brakes on the RAS. This is the raphe system, located in the middle of the RAS. Apparently the raphe system is the chief supplier of the sleep-inducing chemical serotonin, for when cats were surgically deprived of their raphe cells, they became permanent insomniacs and died of exhaustion.

Sleep, the state of consciousness in which man spends a third of his life, was once considered one long cerebral void—seven or eight hours when the brain's circuitry bedded down for unbroken rest; but then a remarkable surge of research in the 1950s revealed sleep to be two distinct states of consciousness. Three quarters of the night is spent in periods of deep relaxation paced by slow, rhythmic brain waves. But four or five times a night, about every 90 minutes, the brain slips into a mysterious second state known as REM sleep, for "rapid eye movement." It was this characteristic that first provided the clue to the existence of the second kind of sleep. In the early 1950s a researcher at the University of Chicago working in a sleep laboratory directed by Nathaniel Kleitman noticed that the eyes of infants darted about rapidly behind closed lids. When the eye movements of adult volunteers were monitored along with their brain waves, Kleitman found a connection. As the eyes began their flickering movements, the brain wave pattern also changed radically. Furthermore, if the volunteers were awakened during REM, they invariably reported that they were dreaming.

From the Chicago laboratory, and from dozens of other sleep research centers in the U.S. and abroad, a detailed portrait of the sleeping brain has emerged. For the first hour or so after the raphe system slows down the RAS to put a man to sleep, he slumbers in comparative peace. A kind of dream may appear, but it is more like a long, rambling thought than the vivid images of REM sleep. The heart rate, blood pressure and breathing begin to slow down during this period, as the brain waves on the EEG machine climb up and down slowly, rhythmically and hypnotically. Some investigators suspect, in fact, that such sleep-inducing stratagems as counting sheep are effective because their rhythms match the slow beat of the brain during early sleep. In laboratories, cats have been put to sleep with similar electrical frequencies.

Occasionally this picture of utter peacefulness is belied by the appearance of quick, jagged peaks on the EEG's graph, showing that the brain's sensory apparatus is still reacting to outside stimuli—a noise, even the touch of the pillow. But ordinarily these signals are too weak to rouse the attention of the brain's alertness system, the RAS, and thus

Labs for picking sleepers' brains

The average person spends a third of his life sleeping, and his brain never stops working during that time. Sleep affords a unique opportunity to study brain functions, and much data comes from tests of sleepers. There is no lack of subjects—an ad for men who slept more than nine hours or fewer than six brought 400 applications.

Observations of sleepers and analyses of their brain waves have produced a string of surprising insights. Depriving people of dreams may threaten their mental stability. Sleepwalking occurs in the deepest sleep, and contrary to the comic strips and movies, people sleepwalk in a normal manner, not with arms outstretched. Normal sleep promotes body growth, but dreaming sleep is needed for growth of the brain.

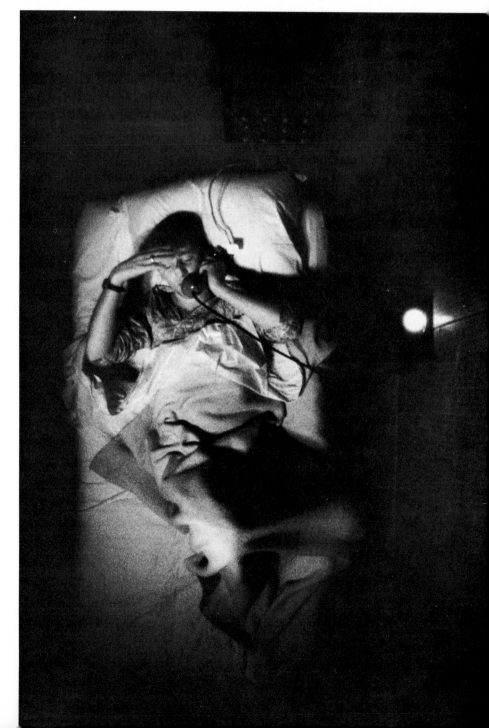

Awakened by a phone call from an observer at a sleep laboratory, a volunteer groggily recounts a dream. Such tests show that dreams vary in length from around 10 minutes to half an hour. About a quarter of the entire night's sleep is taken up by dreaming.

In a series of experiments in extrasensory
perception, one test investigated the
influence of sleep on telepathy. The man
at right below—awake—was directed to
concentrate on a picture and mentally
transmit its image to a girl asleep in
another room (left). When the girl awoke
and was shown the picture along with
three others, she most often picked it as
familiar to her—though she had actually
never seen it before.

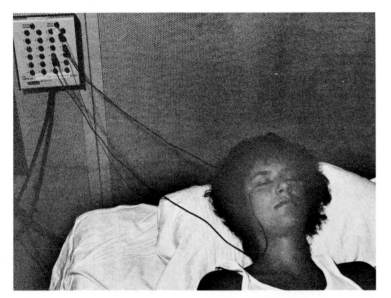

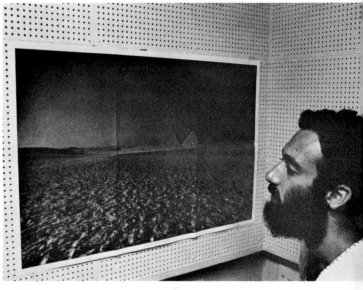

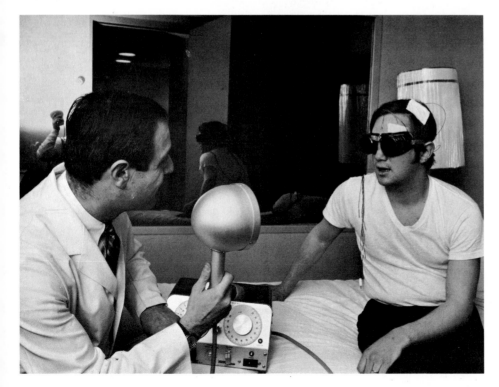

A volunteer wearing red goggles has his
vision checked before going to sleep.
After wearing the goggles for five days,
he dreamed in red. Experiments like this
have demonstrated that experiences while
awake affect dreams in unsuspected ways.
But efforts to make people dream about
particular subjects have failed.

they never reach consciousness. Strangely, the period of slow-wave sleep is the most likely time for bed-wetters or sleepwalkers.

Such activities are the exception, however, for slow-wave sleep is normally a period of tranquil slumber. It ends abruptly when a third mechanism involved in sleep, a cluster of cells above the brain stem called the locus ceruleus ("blue place," because it looks blue)—switches the brain over to REM. Then the synchronous beat of slow-wave sleep is shattered and the EEG records quick, frenetic patterns. The heartbeat quickens too, breathing becomes irregular and the teeth grind. But the neck muscles relax, and this happens so predictably that even in the absence of EEG recordings, it gives away the arrival of REM sleep. Watch someone sleeping in a chair: when the head suddenly slumps forward, the eyes behind their closed lids inevitably begin the flickering movements of REM sleep. The movements literally seem to be following the action of an unfolding dream—the more rapidly the eyes flicker, the more intensely the dreamer participates in his dream. Most of the time the eyes scan from side to side, as they do during wakefulness, but occasionally they move up and down, as the dreamer follows some vertical action. In one experiment, when the dreamer was awakened during a moment of vertical eye movement, he reported dreaming about a small boy who was tossing a ball up and down. Another researcher found that he could often match a dreamer's account of the actions in a dream to the vertical and horizontal eye movements.

The night's first episode of REM sleep lasts only about 10 minutes and yields to another 90 minutes of deep, slow-wave sleep. But each successive period of REM sleep tends to be a little longer than its predecessor. As in wakefulness, the brain seems to concentrate intently during these episodes, but its attention is focused inward rather than on any outside event. Not even a loud noise will produce the distinctive peaks on the EEG that normally signal such intrusions. Internal storm signals do flutter the moving pen occasionally; these are caused by fluctuations in the heart rate, blood pressure and other automatic systems, which seem to be more easily disturbed during REM sleep. These storms increase through the night, and may account for the high frequency of heart attacks in the hours of the early morning.

In one instance REM sleep does not follow its usual cyclical pattern. The bizarre sleeping sickness called narcolepsy bypasses the beginning period of slow-wave sleep and plunges its victims directly into REM. Narcoleptics suffer from overpowering seizures of sleepiness and cannot stay awake. Quite often the urge comes over them when they are emotionally aroused, and they are likely to fall embarassingly asleep in the midst of a funny story, or even while making love.

The discovery that REM sleep is associated with dreaming has opened a new way to study this state of consciousness, so long a subject of mystery and legend. So achingly real yet so alien to the real world of wakefulness, dreams have for millennia served men as a kind of talisman—crystal ball, touchstone on the path to self-knowledge, clue to the inner nature of all things. They have been the raw material for prophesy and foresight since ancient days. They inspired Samuel Taylor Coleridge's poem "Kubla Khan." The German chemist Friedrich Kekulé deciphered the ringlike structure of the carbon atoms in most compounds of living substances after dreaming about a snake devouring its own tail. Sigmund Freud found in dreams the unconscious wishes and drives that are suppressed in waking life, and his disciple Carl Jung believed that dreams contained the grand themes of man's very existence. In addition, the literature of dreams abounds with homelier examples of the insights dreaming provides. For one young man, a dream of red objects arranged in a numerical code supplied the forgotten digits of a girl friend's telephone number.

In the new sleep laboratories the dreams of thousands of volunteers have been observed, and the accumulated data have demolished some long-standing myths. Contrary to popular belief, dreams are not compressed into a few nocturnal moments; they occur in real time—the dream of a half-hour's train ride lasts a half-hour. Some people claim to sleep so soundly they never dream. By morning apparently they have forgotten. For one of the strangest results of the recent sleep research is the discovery of the universality of dreaming. And some evidence indicates that a lack of dreaming may be harmful. When one subject was given drugs to prevent the formation of REM dreams, he began to undergo a change of personality so alarming that the experiment had to be halted after 15 nights. Ordinarily a sober, taciturn man, he suddenly became garrulous and demanded to be taken pub crawling.

A lack of dreaming may also be a factor in the hallucinations and anxieties produced by prolonged wakefulness. One New York disc jockey, who stayed awake for 200 hours as a publicity stunt, claimed he saw a fire in his dresser drawer, spotted a friend's face on a clock dial and fancied that a tweed suit had turned into a mass of furry worms. His delusions occurred every 90 minutes or so, at roughly the intervals when he would normally have been entering a period of REM dreams. Hallucinations, it has been suggested, may compensate for the lost dreams. For REM-deprived sleepers catch up one way or another.

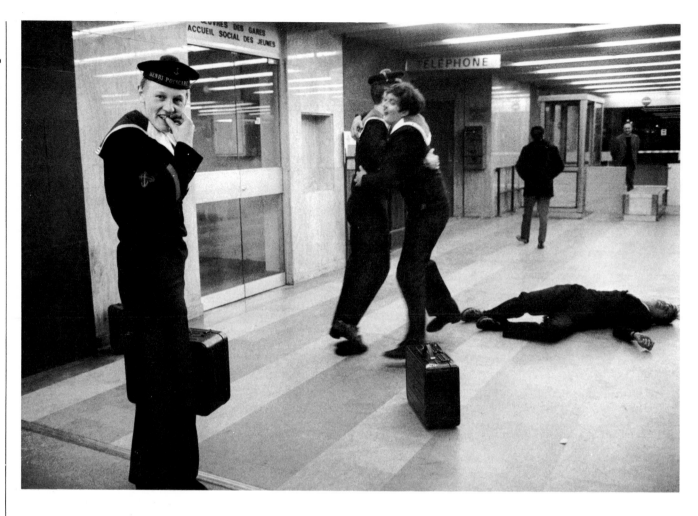

Four French sailors, newly released from service, celebrate in a Paris railway station with an alcohol binge, one of the oldest and commonest ways of altering the mind's state of awareness. Each exhibits effects characteristic of many drugs affecting consciousness: giggly euphoria, uncertain balance and blackout.

People shortchanged on dreams one night automatically dream more often the following night—until they have met their normal quota. Animals do the same thing. Experimenting with cats in 1959, the French physiologist Michel Jouvet used an ingenious technique to keep them from dreaming. He placed his subjects on a low pedestal in a pool of water. Every time the cats went into REM sleep, their neck muscles relaxed and their heads dipped into the water, jarring them into wakefulness. When, after several weeks of dreamlessness, the cats were at last permitted to sleep without interruption, they—just like human volunteers—spent the next few days appeasing their REM hunger. This need to catch up on lost dreaming has also been noted among people who use "uppers" and "downers"—amphetamine energizers and barbiturate sedatives. Although the barbiturates induce sleep, they reduce REM, so that the brain on subsequent nights needs to dream an extra measure to make up. But amphetamines, often taken in the morning to get moving again after drugged slumber, also cut down REM. Thus anyone who regularly takes uppers and downers is embarked on a dangerous cycle of dreamless sleep.

Why dreaming should be so vital is a matter of much conjecture. Sleep obviously is necessary to rest and restore the body's mechanisms, and most scientists believe that this restoration is accomplished during slow-wave sleep. But why did nature dictate a second, different state, and destine man to spend more than a tenth of his life in it?

The most persuasive explanations for dreaming tie it to a process of wearing the brain in, giving its 10 billion nerve cells an opportunity to consolidate the day's learning into long-term memory and adjust to new modes of behavior. In one analogy to computers, the dream is held to be a device for clearing out old programs and debugging new ones. There is evidence for this view in animal studies—monkeys trained to press levers when shown certain images will, after they drift into REM sleep, start pressing the levers again. And some scientists detect this kind of acting out in the dreams of infants. They believe that the REM sleep of a young brain prepares the baby for life by rehearsing him in instinctive behavior. As he dreams he can be seen to suck, smile and exercise his limbs. Indeed, the dreaming infant even shows the beginnings of sexual arousal, which will mark REM sleep throughout adult life. Perhaps the young child's need to learn so much is the reason he dreams so much; the time an infant spends in REM sleep accounts for about half his total sleep of 16 to 18 hours a day, a proportion that gradually tapers off until REM represents only about 13 per cent of sleep.

Among the many other fascinating explanations for dreaming is one making REM sleep an emotional safety valve. According to this theory, dreams allow the individual to go quietly and safely insane every night of his life. By this reckoning mental illness is a kind of misplaced dreaming, switched on by mistake during waking hours. This notion of dreams' function is based on a number of observations: the confused behavior of people deprived of REM sleep; the bouts of insomnia that often precede attacks of mental illness; and the fact that schizophrenics dream less than other people and when deprived of dreams, do not catch up.

The possibility of a connection between dreaming and insanity is strengthened by the new knowledge of the electrochemical processes providing the brain's control of behavior (Chapter 2). Two key compounds known to be involved in sleep are also believed to be essential to mental balance. One of these chemicals is serotonin, the substance that slows down the RAS alertness control; the other is norepinephrine, a substance that accumulates in the locus ceruleus after it has switched the brain to REM sleep. From a variety of clinical and laboratory evidence,

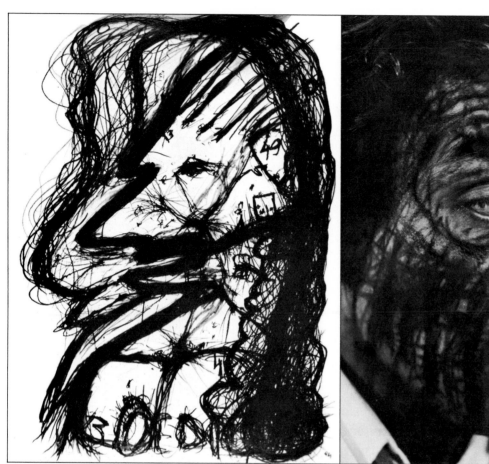

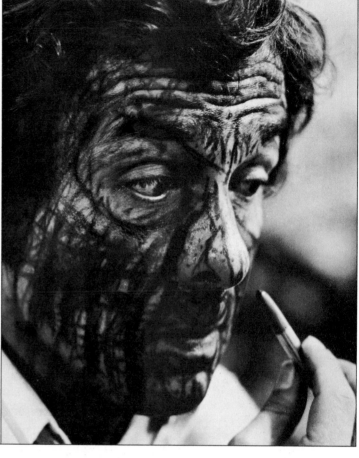

Art that mirrors an altered mind

In 1943 a Swiss chemist named Albert Hofmann accidentally swallowed a tiny amount of the synthetic chemical lysergic acid diethylamide. "There surged upon me," he later wrote, "a stream of fantastic images . . . accompanied by an intense play of colors." Hofmann had discovered the effects of LSD, a potent consciousness-altering drug.

LSD is believed to enhance the activity of norepinephrine and dopamine —chemicals that help to maintain alertness—and also to inhibit the sedative serotonin. The imbalance of these chemicals in the brain produces hallucinations suggestive of insanity.

To test LSD's effect on creativity, 34 artists in Munich took small doses of the drug. Each then studied one of his own works and made another based on it. Their before-and-after efforts show the resemblance between the effects of LSD and those of mental illness.

LSD made Viennese artist Arnulf Rainer turn to a mirror and begin irrationally applying paint to his own face (above), murmuring, "My face becomes like a window picture." Ordinarily he paints portraits like the one at left.

The controlled fantasy of artist Bernhard Jager's piglike animal (near right) disintegrated under LSD into the sketch at the far right, which he drew with difficulty, complaining, "Everything begins to move in this picture."

Peter Collier is noted for the precise draftsmanship of his surrealist anatomical studies (below). But after taking LSD he drew a vague sketch of a more bloated female form (right).

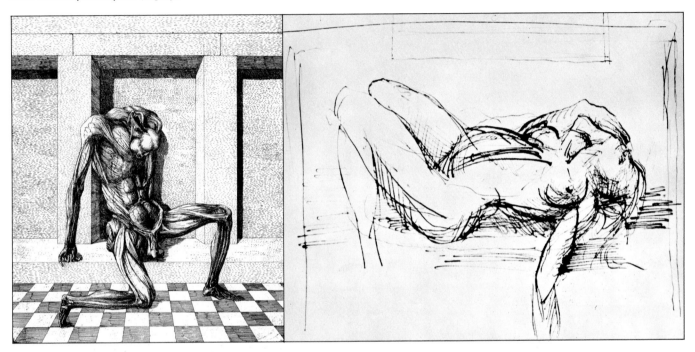

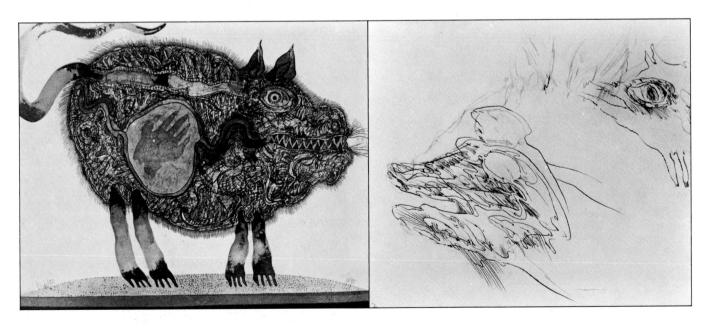

it appears that too much or too little of either of these substances may be a factor in madness. Though the picture is incomplete and the puzzle far from solved, some scientists believe that one day aberrant behavior will be corrected by chemically retuning the brain's nerve circuits.

At the moment no one can consciously control the mechanisms in the brain that bring on sleep or wakefulness and that affect the progress of insanity. Often a sufferer from severe mental illness can be observed switching inexorably into psychosis; his behavior turns abruptly from rational to irrational and he is unable to prevent the change. Yet it now appears that the brain has more power to control its actions than anyone had guessed. Normal activities of the nervous system that had seemed entirely automatic—regulation of heart rate and blood pressure, for example—can apparently be altered at will. Some experiments have produced astonishing results. Sufferers from high blood pressure have been taught to reduce their abnormal pressures by an act of will. Victims of migraine—severe headaches associated with the expansion of certain blood vessels—have learned to recognize the symptoms of an oncoming attack and then consciously prevent the blood vessels from expanding. It is as though the brain can learn to bring up to a conscious level some actions that ordinarily are unconscious.

The process of learning to control the uncontrollable is called biofeedback training. It involves informing an individual of what is going on inside his brain so that he can govern its operations.

The earliest research into biofeedback training focused on the brain's alpha waves—the rhythmic patterns associated with the daydreaming state—and was conducted in 1958 at the University of Chicago's sleep laboratory. A young psychologist, Joe Kamiya, became intrigued with the way his sleep volunteers seemed able to guess their brains had slipped into the long, leisurely patterns of the alpha rhythm. Following this lead, he was amazed to discover that the volunteers could turn on their alpha waves at will, although the shift into the alpha state is normally automatic and unfelt. He put his subjects in a darkened soundproof room, fastened electrodes on their scalps feeding into an EEG machine, and whenever they produced an alpha wave, he gave them a kind of reward—a pleasant musical tone. Within a few hours the subjects became masters of the new art of governing levels of consciousness. But unfortunately they were never quite certain how the mastery was attained—except that it was not done by trying. Indeed, when they concentrated on making alpha waves, they produced nothing but the beta waves of the alert state. Only when they gave up trying did the alpha waves appear.

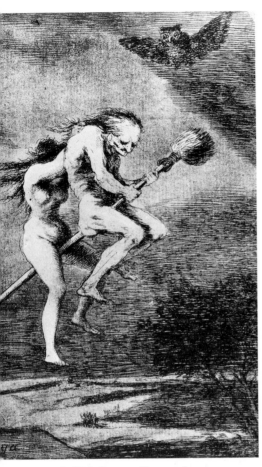

In 17th Century Europe there were women who claimed to be witches and insisted they could fly, like the witches in this Goya etching. They apparently believed this, but the contemporary French physician Jean de Nyauld suggested that their flights were imaginary, induced by rubbing the body with hallucinogenic ointments to alter the consciousness.

Soon after Kamiya's discovery a second avenue of biofeedback research led to mastery over the visceral responses such as heartbeat, blood pressure and skin temperature. Controlled by muscles that take their orders from a command center deep within the brain, the hypothalamus, these functions were long thought to be wholly involuntary. Messages move to them along the autonomous nervous system, a network of nerves independent of those that serve the voluntary muscles, and until recently no one believed that the autonomous nervous system could be consciously controlled. Eastern mystics who claimed they could slow down their heartbeats or lower their skin temperatures were assumed to be using their voluntary muscles in some subtle fashion to overturn the normal behavior of the visceral muscles.

Then, in the early 1960s, Neal Miller of The Rockefeller University decided to test the autonomous nervous system and see how independent it really was. The technique he devised for his experiment was both ingenious and bizarre: he proposed to teach rats how to change heart rate and blood pressure by expanding and contracting their blood vessels. In order to prevent them from "cheating" by using voluntary chest muscles to effect heartbeat, he paralysed those muscles—but then, since the chest muscles are necessary for breathing, he fitted each rat with a tiny respirator. To encourage the animals in their new tasks, he offered them an electronic reward: a jolt in their pleasure centers whenever they succeeded. Although his results are debated by some scientists, Miller himself was satisfied that the rats did indeed learn a measure of internal control. In fact, one of Miller's students, Leo V. DiCara, reported that one rat became so adept at controlling its blood flow that it could blush in one ear at a time.

Since that initial experiment, biofeedback laboratories have proliferated, and Miller and other biofeedback researchers say they have taught human volunteers to gain at least some mastery over their autonomous nervous systems. Some people have learned to lower their blood pressure and regulate an erratic heartbeat, while others have relieved tension and migraine headache by increasing the flow of blood to their hands—instead of their aching heads. In one experiment, eight victims of cardiac arrhythmia—irregular heartbeat that can be fatal—were taught to stabilize their heart rates. Each patient was informed of his heart rhythm by being connected to a device that controlled colored lights; they flashed red when the rate was abnormally slow, green when too fast and yellow when normal. Five of the eight succeeded in correcting rate variations, forcing their hearts to beat slower or faster to keep the yellow light on. One said he speeded up his heart by turning

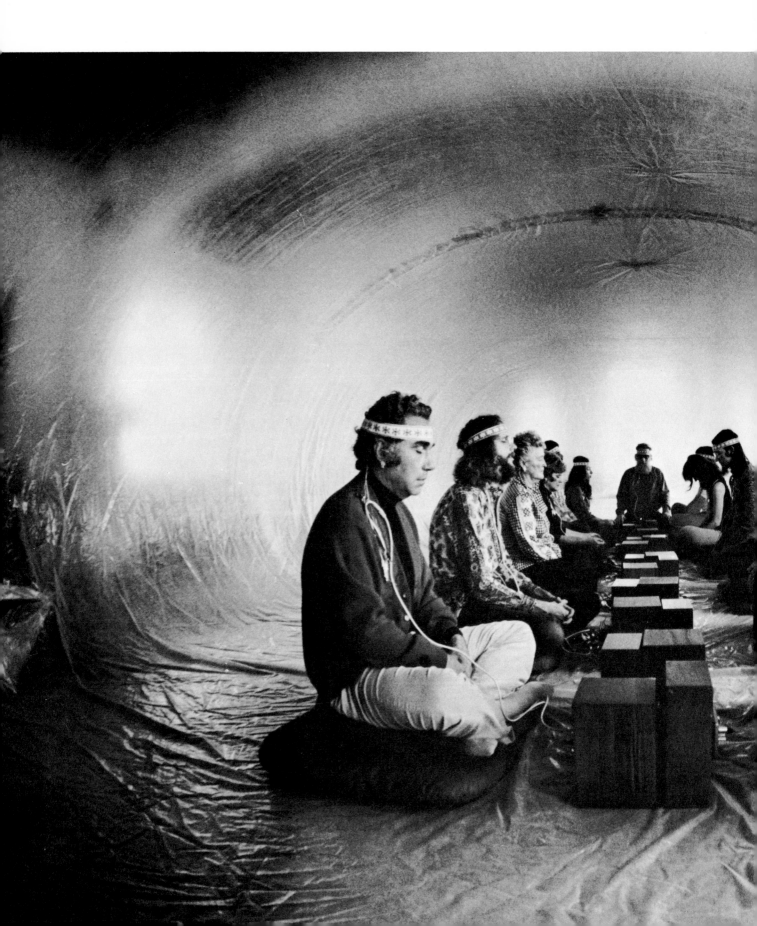

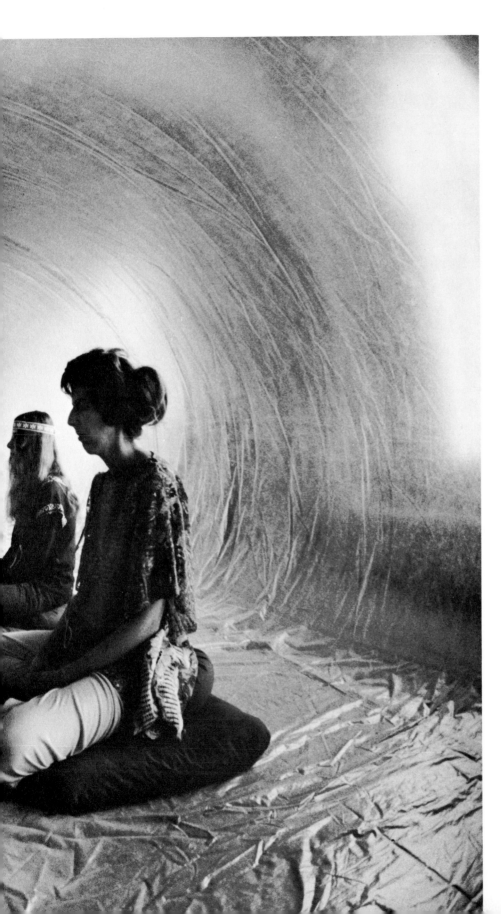

Searching for serenity in the seclusion of an inflated plastic bubble, a group of Californians tries to produce the calm brain waves of the alpha rhythm —characteristic of a state between sleep and wakefulness—on the electronic monitoring machines to which they are attached. Though everyone generates alpha waves when relaxed or slightly drowsy, and Eastern mystics are able to produce them at will, many people learn to attain them more easily with the help of brain-wave instruments.

his mind to a boy bouncing a rubber ball; another increased her rate by thinking about arguing with her children or running on a dark street; and a third slowed her heart rate by imagining she was swinging back and forth on a swing.

Such results have raised hopes of remedying a number of brain-related ills, from insomnia to epilepsy. Some brain-wave researchers are teaching people to produce the soothing rhythms of alpha waves. Others are studying what they believe to be a separate state of consciousness associated with problem solving and creativity. One study of the learning patterns of rats suggests that the so-called theta brain waves, at 4 to 7 cycles per second occurring between deep sleep and dreaming, may signal the brain's readiness to process memories.

More than any other field of brain research, biofeedback has caught the public fancy. Part of its appeal lies in its use of electronic gadgetry. People are intrigued by the notion of being hooked into instruments that enable them to observe variations in their own heartbeats, skin temperatures and brain waves. In addition, some biofeedback machines are set up to provide "rewards" of flashing lights and electronic beeps that make them as much fun to operate as a pinball machine in a penny arcade. In a few cases the rewards are even more novel. In one biofeedback arrangement, a subject's amplified alpha waves set a toy train in motion; in another, a volunteer's control of his heartbeat won him a peep-show glimpse of a pinup.

But it is the potential applications of biofeedback training that excite the most serious interest. Some possibilities have an aura of science fiction. Enthusiasts envision a day when the daydreaming pleasures of alpha-wave breaks will replace coffee breaks; when music imagined by composers will be recorded directly off an EEG machine; when tuned-in lovers will flirt by means of subtle changes in their cerebral voltages. Inevitably, this kind of thinking has turned biofeedback into something of a fad. Entrepreneurs peddle inexpensive, and inaccurate, EEG machines that can be used in the living room to monitor alpha waves, and offer courses in alpha-wave production that promise instant serenity. Yet there are also significant, very productive uses of biofeedback training to be explored. For it offers a way to treat serious illnesses without drugs. No one undervalues the possibility that sufferers from a variety of circulatory ailments—and possibly other diseases—can relieve both symptoms and physical defect by consciously willing the brain to do so.

Biofeedback has also given a kind of scientific credibility to Eastern mysticism. Practitioners of yoga and similar meditation techniques have demonstrated under laboratory conditions that they can switch into the alpha state at will and exercise control over some of their visceral functions. Their ability is apparently based on a quirk in the brain's mechanism for staying alert: the state of awareness requires a constantly changing input of sensory material. Most techniques for meditation deprive the alertness center of this stimulus. The practitioner is required to concentrate on a single object for a long period of time, or even to focus the mind's eye on an internal image. As the result of such intense visual concentration the brain switches off the beta waves of alertness and subsides into alpha rhythms. In one experiment, biofeedback volunteers were fitted with special lenses hooked up to a tiny projector that permitted them to see a single image only, no matter where they moved their eyes. Faced with this unchanging image, they found in time that the image seemed to disappear—and just at the moment it vanished, alpha waves appeared on the EEG machine.

In another inquiry into the use of meditation techniques to influence visceral responses, researchers monitored a group of followers of Maharishi Mahesh Yogi, a teacher of "transcendental meditation." The Maharishi's technique requires the practitioner to focus his attention on a *mantra*—a series of mellifluous words that are repeated silently. The *mantras* did indeed evince a variety of changes in the subjects. The production of alpha waves became more pronounced, the heartbeat slowed, and the body decreased its production of blood lactate—a substance associated with anxiety. In fact, in purely physiological terms, the meditative state produced symptoms that were exactly opposite to those produced during states of stress. And since stress responses are suspected of being the source of many illnesses, some biofeedback researchers are suggesting that meditation—or biofeedback training —may become an important tool in the prevention and cure of such typically modern ailments as hypertension and ulcers.

The current fascination with the use of biofeedback training and Eastern mysticism to probe the mysteries of the human mind is of course greeted with skepticism by many brain scientists. Alpha waves and autonomic control seem light-years away from the patient, painstaking attempts to fathom how the brain's 10 billion nerve cells convert simple electrical impulses into the myriad complexities of human behavior. Still, the very idea of self-control is refreshing. After all the brave-new-world tinkering with the brain through drugs, electric currents and surgery, it is rather pleasant to contemplate the return to a tradition as old as the one that holds the human brain has the power both to understand and to transcend itself.

Seeking the limits of the mind

In a single 24-hour period, almost everyone will experience four states of consciousness: full wakefulness; daydreaming, or reverie; deep, dreamless sleep, and the sleep of dreams. Almost everyone, too, has witnessed or experienced a fifth state—the altered consciousness of alcohol intoxication. Less common are states of consciousness produced by drugs, hypnosis and meditation. In these states, brain waves shift in pattern. Hallucinations replace reality. Individuals become insensitive to pain, or perform superhuman feats.

Scientists have found no firm explanations of the mechanisms at work when consciousness is changed. While they accumulate evidence and test hypotheses, thousands of people around them deliberately seek out altered states of consciousness. Some use drugs—intoxicants like marijuana or hallucinogens like LSD. Others attain trancelike states in repetitive, autohypnotic chants and dances. Still others follow the disciplines of meditation.

Many of these modern seekers of altered awareness insist that, in changing their own lives, they also make contact with older cultural traditions. In one sense, at least, they are quite correct. Almost every road to altered states of consciousness has been explored and traveled by other cultures. The Barasana Indians of the upper Amazon use coca—the raw material of cocaine—to stimulate pious trances. The dervishes of the Middle East and the Balinese of the Far East change consciousness by dancing; the followers of yoga by meditation. Such groups seek altered states of awareness for other worldly revelations, for the welfare of a tribe—or, occasionally, just for fun.

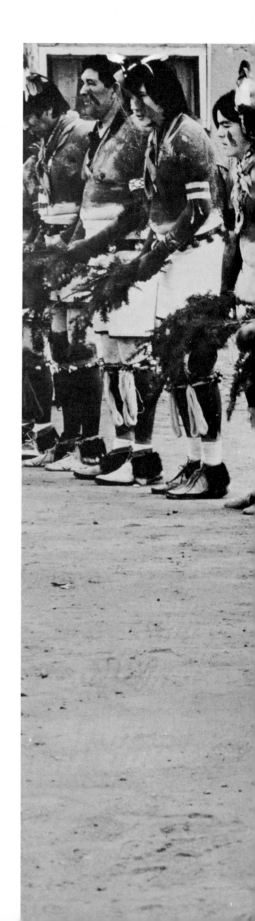

The day-long Cloud Dance of New Mexico's San Juan Indians, performed in January or February, invokes a successful year for the tribe. Each dancer concentrates his mental energy on the hypnotic rhythm of the dance, finally reaching a point at which he is unaware of the intense midwinter cold.

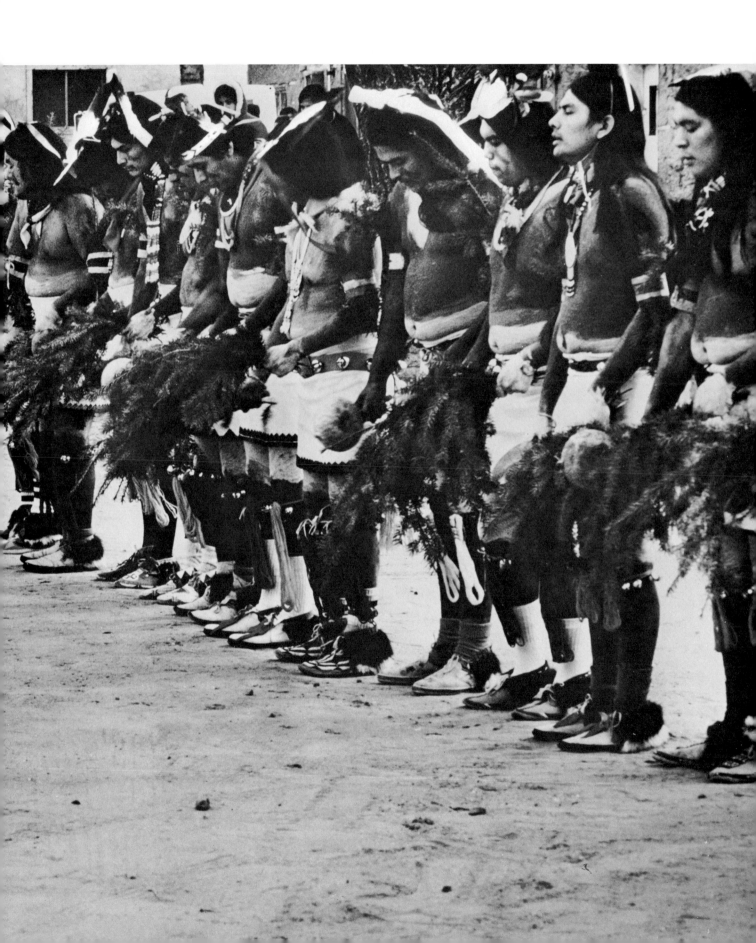

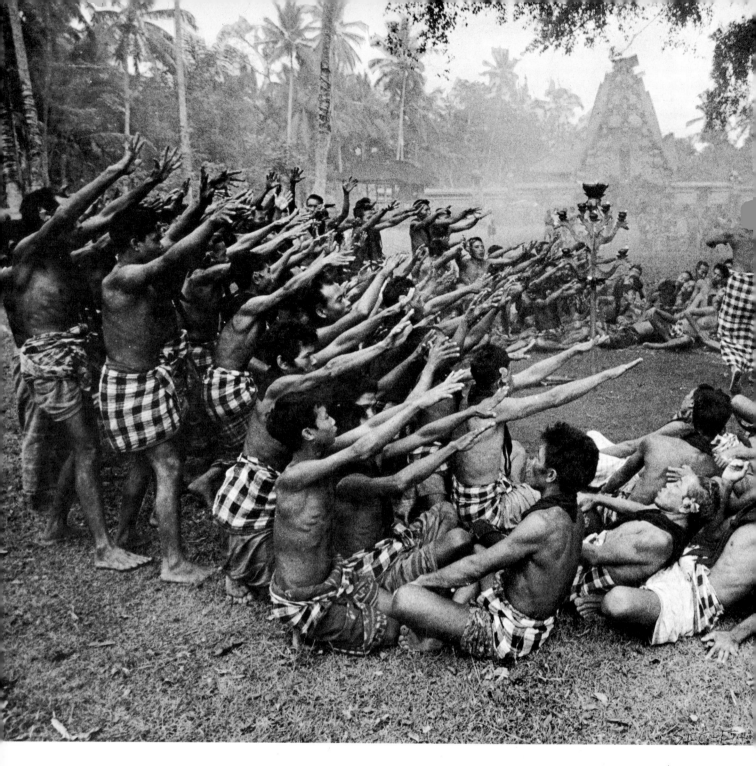

The trancelike dances of Bali

Dance is an integral part of Bali's religion. Long, complex tales of gods and goddesses are enacted in dance against a background of temple walls, before sacred banyan trees and even in secular gatherings, but the dancers are never mere entertainers. As good wins out over evil, wicked spirits founder, and heroes and gods triumph in the pattern of the dance, the dancers themselves undergo profound changes in consciousness: hypnotized by their own chants and movements, they enter upon a religious experience marked by trancelike states and extraordinary feats of agility and precision.

Every village has its own orchestra and dance troupe that regularly join together for religious performances. One of the most popular is the Ketjak Dance, shown here, which relates an episode in the life of the Hindu god Rama.

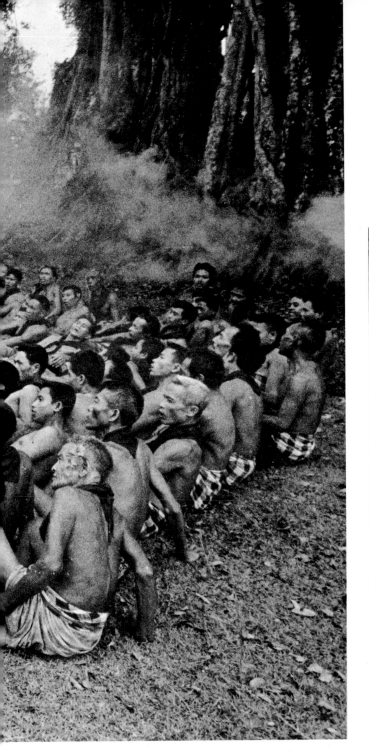

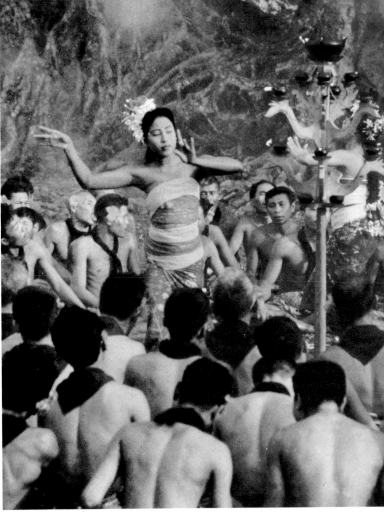

Rhythmically throwing their arms forward, then back, and shouting, "tjak, tjak, tjak!" in imitation of a troupe of angry monkeys, Balinese villagers play the part of a victorious monkey army rushing to help the god Rama rescue his kidnapped wife in the Ketjak Dance.

A young Balinese girl takes one of the central roles in the Ketjak. Like many of the villagers seated around her, she is in a self-induced trance that will enable her to perform rapid and intricate measures without errors or fatigue.

163

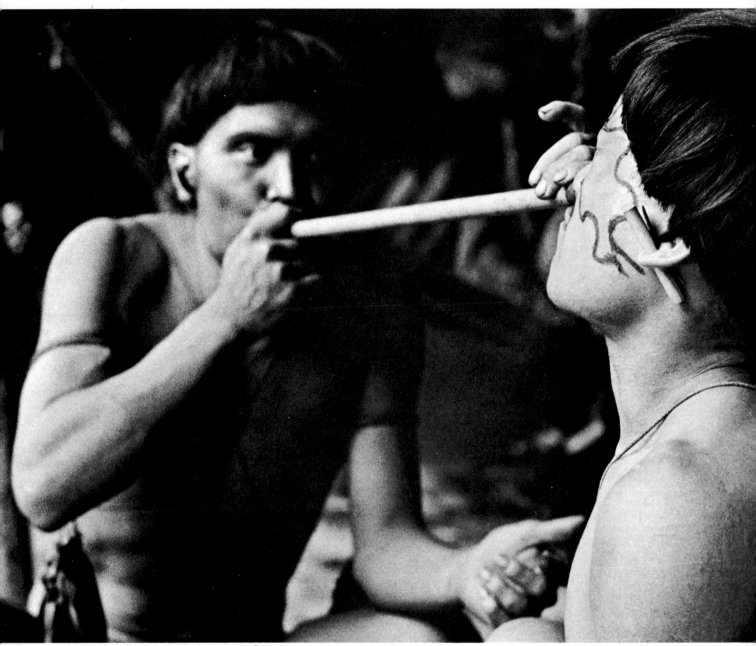

A Yanomamö uses a hollow tube to blow powdered ebene directly into a companion's nostrils. The drug will take effect moments later.

A drug that unleashes violence

For the Yanomamö Indians of northern Brazil and Venezuela, drugs sometimes create alterations of awareness—and behavior so violent that they erupt into bloodshed. Before a tribal feast the Yanomamös inhale the powdered bark of the *ebene* tree. Under the influence of this hallucinogenic drug, they engage in ceremonial duels in which they mercilessly pound one another's chests; if the combatants come from potentially hostile villages or hold personal grudges, the duels can escalate into pitched battles. But the Yanomamö also use the *ebene* drug for peaceful purposes: to exorcize evil spirits from the sick; to stimulate the spirit of affection and even of cooperation between neighboring tribes—or what passes for cooperation in a fierce, competitive people—and, now and then, simply to relax at the end of a day.

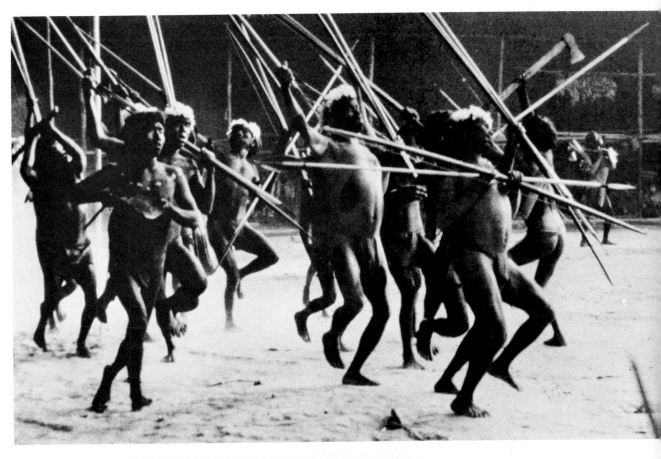

Intoxicated with ebene, Yanomamö men dance around their village, preparing for a formal chest-pounding duel. Some carry tubes to administer the drug, some brandish weapons, and the man at left holds a piece of a vessel in which ebene bark was ground to a powder.

These two men danced in the parade shown above, then pounded each other's chests. Now, still under the influence of the drug, they chant blearily but affectionately about all kinds of future friendships and alliances.

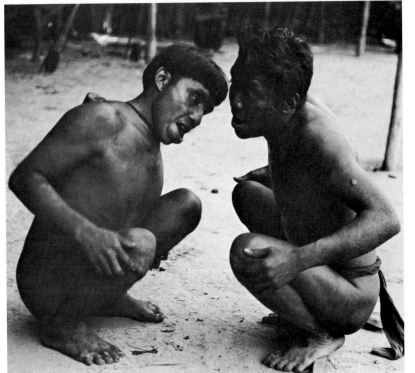

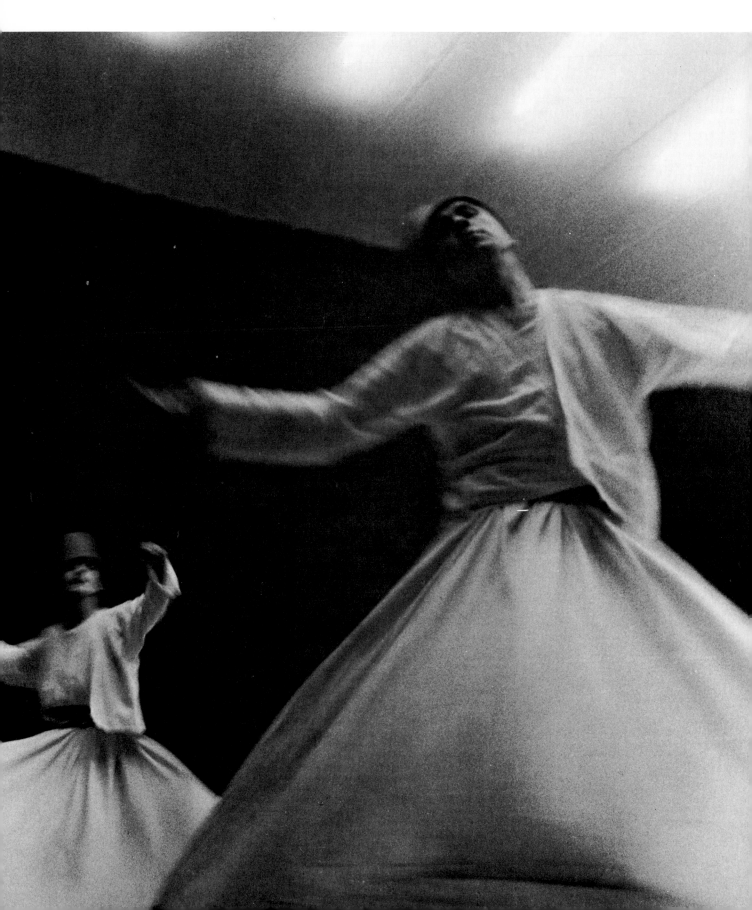

The ecstasies
of the dervishes

Over 800 years ago, a group of Muslim ascetics founded Sufism, a sect which is devoted to achieving a union of the worshipper with God. Some descendants, notably the Qadiris of Kurdistan and the Maulavis of Turkey, survive as dervishes (a Persian word for beggar). Like all Muslims, dervishes worship Allah—but their rituals go beyond the usual prayers and fasting into altered states of consciousness. Both Maulavis and Qadiris consider the world to be a tomb or a prison for the soul, separating it from Allah. To reunite their souls with God, the Qadiris chant for hours till they enter into a trance. With their normal consciousness suspended, they are able to perform startling acts of faith—piercing their cheeks, handling deadly snakes, touching red-hot metal. The Maulavis, the famous "whirling" dervishes, spin in a religious transport to the accompaniment of flutes and drums, convinced that their souls join Allah for the length of the dance.

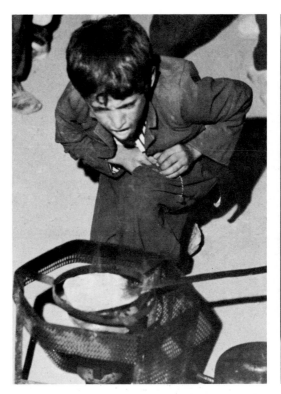 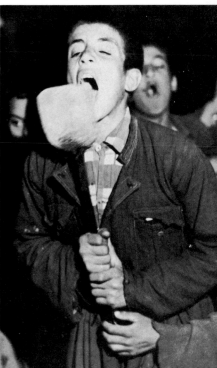

Circling majestically, Turkish dervishes worship God in an endless, hypnotic whirl. The dancers insist that the dance is calm and controlled. "It is a spiritual thing," says one dervish. "We don't give ourselves over to unreality."

A Qadiri boy chants over a red-hot poker (left) as he goes into a trance that blocks pain. Meanwhile, another Qadiri touches a hot poker to his tongue (right). Said one child: "I shout out to God and he takes away the pain. Otherwise, I'd die."

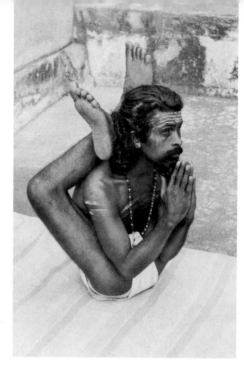

A practitioner of hatha-yoga, a Hindu spiritual and physical discipline, locks his body into a deeply contorted posture as he directs his mind toward the deity (right). Similar yoga exercises control breathing, blood flow and other normally involuntary processes.

Mesmerized by meditation

Most religions incorporate some form of meditation and all techniques of meditation are basically similar, though they may seem different. Hindus chant semimelodic syllables. Zen monks puzzle over paradoxes such as "What is the sound of one hand clapping?" Kalahari Bushmen gaze fixedly at the moon. All of these actions call for intense concentration on a single sound, thought or object to the exclusion of all else. With normal outside stimuli eliminated, the brain's focus shifts to a more internal state of consciousness.

The purpose behind the shift varies: for the Hindu ascetics shown on these pages, the object of meditation is union with a deity; for secular Westerners, it may be deliberate control of such normally involuntary processes as heartbeat *(page 154)*. But all human beings, from the Bushmen to big-city inhabitants, have essentially the same nervous system, and all use similar means to reach altered states of consciousness.

A form of yoga-like discipline is demonstrated by a sadhu, or holy man (left), who lies in a trance on a bed of sharp cactus spines, oblivious to pain in the depth of his meditation.

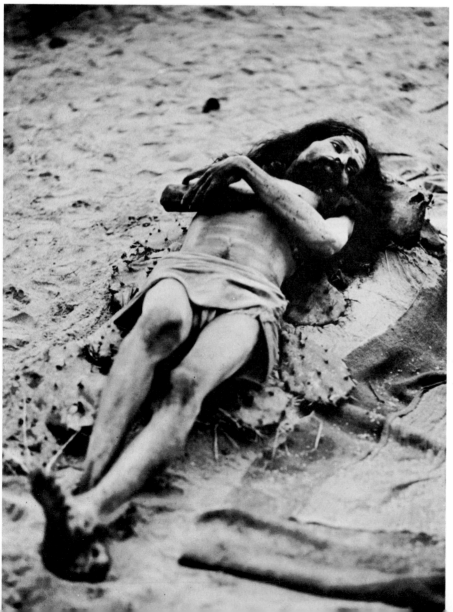

At the headwaters of the Ganges, a holy river, two sadhus meditate (right), concentrating on the monotonous river sound. Said one, "I slowly forget my surroundings . . . I am like a child."

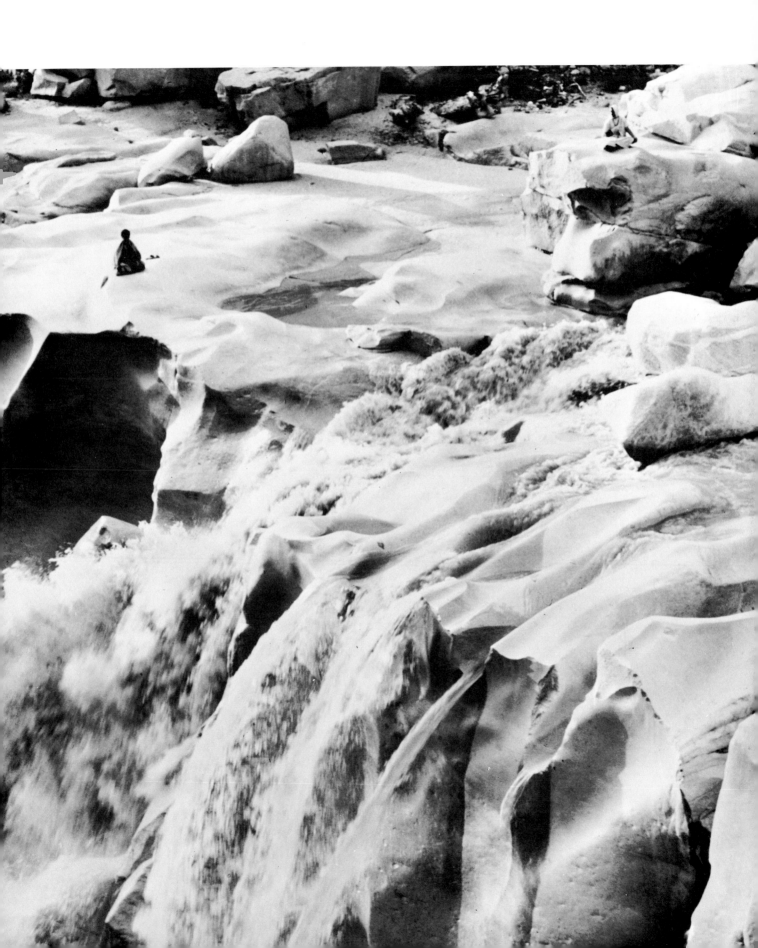

Bibliography

Books

Atkinson, Richard C., ed., *Contemporary Psychology*. W. H. Freeman & Co., 1971.

Brown, Barbara B., *New Mind, New Body*. Harper & Row, Publishers, 1974.

Calder, Nigel, *The Mind of Man*. The Viking Press, 1973.

Chagnon, Napoleon A.:
Studying the Yanomamö. Holt, Rinehart and Winston, 1974.
Yanomamö, The Fierce People. Holt, Rinehart and Winston, 1968.

Chalmers, Neil, Roberta Crawley and Steven P. R. Rose, eds., *The Biological Bases of Behavior*. Harper & Row, Publishers, 1971.

Eccles, John C., *The Understanding of the Brain*. McGraw-Hill Book Co., 1973.

Ferguson, Marilyn, *The Brain Revolution: The Frontiers of Mind Research*. Taplinger Publishing Co., 1973.

Ford, Donald, and J. P. Schadé, *Atlas of the Human Brain*. Elsevier Publishing Co., 1966.

Galambos, Robert, *Nerves and Muscles*. Doubleday & Co., 1962.

Gazzaniga, Michael S., *The Bisected Brain*. Appleton-Century-Crofts, 1970.

Gregory, R. L.:
Eye and Brain: The Psychology of Seeing. McGraw-Hill Book Co., 1966.
The Intelligent Eye. McGraw-Hill Book Co., 1970.

Grossman, Sebastian P., *Essentials of Physiological Psychology*. John Wiley & Sons, 1973.

Harner, Michael J., ed., *Hallucinogens and Shamanism*. Oxford University Press, 1973.

Jonas, Gerald, *Visceral Learning: Toward a Science of Self-Control*. The Viking Press, 1973.

Kimber, Diana Clifford, Carolyn E. Gray and Caroline E. Stackpole, *Anatomy and Physiology*. The Macmillan Co., 1966.

Lausch, Erwin, *Manipulation: Dangers and Benefits of Brain Research*. The Viking Press, 1974.

Lawrence, Jodi, *Alpha Brain Waves*. Nash Publishing, 1972.

Lowenstein, Otto, *The Senses*. Penguin Books, 1966.

Luria, A. R., *The Mind of a Mnemonist*. Translated from the Russian by Lynn Solotaroff. Basic Books, 1968.

Mark, Vernon H., and Frank R. Ervin, *Violence and the Brain*. Harper & Row, Publishers, 1970.

Nilsson, Lennart, *Behold Man*. Little, Brown & Co., 1973.

Noback, Charles R., and Robert J. Demarest, *The Nervous System*. McGraw-Hill Book Co., 1972.

Ornstein, Robert E.:
ed., *The Nature of Human Consciousness*. The Viking Press, 1974.
The Psychology of Consciousness. The Viking Press, 1972.

Penfield, W., and T. Rasmussen, *The Cerebral Cortex of Man*. The Macmillan Co., 1950.

Pincus, Jonathan H., and Gary Tucker, *Behavioral Neurology*. Oxford University Press, 1974.

Pines, Maya, *The Brain Changers*. Harcourt Brace Jovanovich, 1973.

Plutchik, Robert, *Emotions: Facts, Theories, and a New Model*. Random House, 1962.

Pribram, K. H., ed., *Brain and Behaviour*, 4 Vols. Penguin Books, 1969.

Robbins, Rossell Hope, *The Encyclopedia of Witchcraft and Demonology*. Crown Publishers, 1959.

Rose, Steven, *The Conscious Brain*. Alfred A. Knopf, 1973.

Stevens, Leonard A., *Explorers of the Brain*. Alfred A. Knopf, 1971.

Truex, Raymond C., and Malcolm B. Carpenter, *Human Neuroanatomy*, 6th ed. The Williams & Wilkins Co., 1969.

U.S. Department of Health, Education and Welfare, *Current Research on Sleep and Dreams*. Public Health Service Publication No. 1389.

Valenstein, Elliot S., *Brain Control: A Critical Examination of Brain Stimulation and Psychosurgery*. John Wiley & Sons, 1973.

Weil, Andrew, *The Natural Mind*. Houghton Mifflin Co., 1972.

Wilentz, Joan Steen, *The Senses of Man*. Thomas Y. Crowell Co., 1969.

Wooldridge, Dean E., *The Machinery of the Brain*. McGraw-Hill Book Co., 1963.

Zangwill, O. L., *Cerebral Dominance and its Relation to Psychological Functions*. Oliver and Boyd, 1960.

Periodicals

Agranoff, Bernard W., "Memory and Protein Synthesis." *Scientific American* (June 1967), pp. 115-122.

Axelrod, Julius, "Neurotransmitters." *Scientific American* (June 1974), pp. 59-71.

Bizzi, Emilio, "The Coordination of Eye-Head Movements." *Scientific American* (October 1974), pp. 100-106.

Ceraso, John, "The Interference Theory of Forgetting." *Scientific American* (October 1967), pp. 117-124.

Evarts, Edward V., "Brain Mechanisms in Movement." *Scientific American* (July 1973); pp. 96-103.

Fisher, Alan E., "Chemical Stimulation of the Brain." *Scientific American* (June 1964), pp. 60-68.

Gazzaniga, Michael S., "The Split Brain in Man." *Scientific American* (August 1967), pp. 24-29.

Gerard, Ralph W., "What is Memory?" *Scientific American* (September 1953), pp. 118-126.

Geschwind, Norman, "Language and the Brain." *Scientific American* (April 1972), pp. 76-83.

Gross, Charles G., C. E. Rocha-Miranda and D. B. Bender, "Visual Properties of Neurons in Inferotemporal Cortex of the Macaque." *Journal of Neurophysiology*, Vol. XXXV, No. 1 (1972).

Guillemin, Roger, and Roger Burgus, "The Hormones of the Hypothalamus." *Scientific American* (November 1972), pp. 24-33.

Haber, Ralph Norman, "Eidetic Images." *Scientific American* (April 1969), pp. 36-44.

Heimer, Lennart, "Pathways in the Brain." *Scientific American* (July 1971), pp. 48-60.

Hubel, David H., "The Visual Cortex of the Brain." *Scientific American* (November 1963), pp. 54-55.

Jouvet, Michel, "The States of Sleep." *Scientific American* (February 1967), pp. 62-72.

Kimura, Doreen, "The Asymmetry of the Human Brain." *Scientific American* (March 1973), pp. 70-78.

Levine, Seymour, "Sex Differences in the Brain." *Scientific American* (April 1966), pp. 84-90.

Llinas, Rodolfo R., "The Cortex of the Cerebellum." *Scientific American* (January 1975), pp. 56-71.

Merton, P. A., "How We Control the Contraction of Our Muscles." *Scientific American* (May 1972), pp. 30-37.

Michael, Charles R., "Retinal Processing of Visual Images." *Scientific American* (May 1969), pp. 104-114.

Oster, Gerald, "Auditory Beats in the Brain." *Scientific American* (October 1973), pp. 94-102.

Penfield, Wilder, "The Uncommitted Cortex: The Child's Changing Brain." *Scientific American* (July 1964), pp. 77-81.

Pribram, Karl H., "The Neurophysiology of Remembering." *Scientific American* (January 1969), pp. 73-86.

Richards, Whitman, "The Fortification Illusions of Migraines." *Scientific American* (May 1971), pp. 88-96.

Rosensweig, Mark R., Edward L. Bennett and Marian C. Diamond, "Brain Changes in Response to Experience." *Scientific American* (February 1972), pp. 22-29.

Snider, Ray S., "The Cerebellum." *Scientific American* (August 1958), pp. 84-90.

Sperry, Roger W., "The Great Cerebral Commissure." *Scientific American* (January 1964), pp. 42-52.

Wurtman, Richard J., and Julius Axelrod, "The Pineal Gland." *Scientific American* (July 1965), pp. 50-60.

Acknowledgments

The author and editors of this book are particularly indebted to Saran Jonas, M.D., Associate Professor of Clinical Neurology, New York University School of Medicine, New York City, and Michael S. Gazzaniga, Department of Psychology, State University of New York, Stony Brook, New York. They also wish to thank the following persons and institutions: Judith, Nathan, Ruth and Esme Farb, New York City; Mrs. Charles Stewart Flagg, New York City; Donald Hood, Associate Professor, Department of Psychology, Columbia University, New York City; Robert E. Ornstein, Department of Medical Psychology, University of California Medical Center, San Francisco, California; Fred Schwartz, Director of Internship Training, New York Hospital, Westchester Division; Leon Sternfeld, M.D., Medical Director, United Cerebral Palsy Association, Inc.

Picture Credits

Sources for illustrations (credits from left to right are separated by semicolons, from top to bottom by dashes):

Cover—Norman Snyder. 6—Duane Michals. 9—The Bettmann Archive. 11—The Bettmann Archive; Radio Times Hulton. 15—Douglas Faulkner—Edward S. Ross. 16—Dan Budnik from Woodfin Camp and Associates—Eliot Elisofon, courtesy Eliot Elisofon estate. 17—John Dominis from TIME-LIFE Picture Agency—Nina Leen. 19, 21—Drawings by Jim Alexander. 22—Michael Mauney. 25—Lola Goujon. 26—Earl Dotter from BBM. Drawings pages 30 through 42 by Jim Alexander. 30, 31—Pål-Nils Nilsson from Tio. 32, 33—Martti Brandt from Suomen Kuvapalvelu; Christian and Margaret Murray. 34—Anthony Wolff. 35—Ken Regan from Camera 5. 36, 37—Manfred Vollmer; Fred Lyon from Rapho Guillumette. 38—George Krause. 39—Mitchell Payne from Jeroboam. 40, 41—Henri Cartier-Bresson; © Leo Touchet. 42, 43—Jerry Cooke. 44—Dan Bernstein. 49—Lennart Nilsson. 50—Lennart Nilsson; Lennart Nilsson, from *Behold Man*, published by Little, Brown and Co., Boston 1974. 51, 52—Lennart Nilsson, from *Behold Man*, published by Little, Brown and Co., Boston 1974. 57—Walter Scheiwiller. 60—From *Language of Vision* by Gyorgy Kepes, published by Paul Theobald and Co., 1944. 62—Ron James; Jay Dorin. 64—Graham Finlayson. 66 through 77—Nathan Farb. 78—Henri Dauman. 81—Drawing by Jim Alexander, adapted from "The Split Brain in Man" by Michael S. Gazzaniga. © August 1967 by *Scientific American*. All rights reserved. 83—Ross Loos Medical Group. 85—Michael S. Gazzaniga. 86, 87—Philip Daly. 88, 89—B. P. Grimaud. 92—Ernst Haas. 96, 97—Associated Newspapers. 101 through 104—Melissa Shook. 108—David Powers from Jeroboam. 112—Ellen Pines from Woodfin Camp and Associates. 115—Les Wilson from Camera Press. 117—Bill Binzen. 118—Alan Mercer. 121—Terry Fincher, *London Express*. 123—John Loengard from TIME-LIFE Picture Agency. 125—Elek Toth. 128, 129—Brian Seed. 130, 131—James Karales. 132—Thomas Höpker from Woodfin Camp and Associates. 133—Brian Seed from Black Star. 134, 135—Bert Stern; Al Francekevich. 136—James Karales. 137—Ron Burton from Syndication International. 138—Joanne Leonard. 142, 143—*National Enquirer*. 145—Gazette Photo Service. 146—Ralph Morse from TIME-LIFE Picture Agency. 147—Marcia Keegan, courtesy Psi SEARCH exhibition produced for California Museum of Science and Industry in cooperation with Parapsychological Association—Ken Heyman. 150—Guy Le Querrec/VIVA from Woodfin Camp and Associates. 152—Friedrich Rauch; Albert Ammer. 153—Friedrich Rauch except upper left Peter Collien. 155—Nina Leen. 156, 157—Ralph Crane from TIME-LIFE Picture Agency. 160, 161—Marcia Keegan. 162, 163—Thomas Höpker from Woodfin Camp and Associates. 164, 165—Napoleon Chagnon. 166—Dave Bellak from Jeroboam. 167—Granada Television. 168—Süddeutscher Verlag—Raghubir Singh from Woodfin Camp and Associates. 169—Raghubir Singh from Woodfin Camp and Associates.

Index

Numerals in italics indicate a photograph or drawing of the subject mentioned.

A

Acetylcholine, 54
Adrenal gland, 120, 121
Adrenal hormones: epinephrine as, 120; functions of, 120; norepinephrine as, 120, 121; order for release of, 120; parallel release of, 120-121; source of, 120
Aggression, 110, 124, *130-131*; center of, 114-115; influence of hypothalamus on, 119
Agranoff, Bernard, 99
Albertus Magnus, 9; conception of brain of, *9*
Alcohol, 29; alteration of state of awareness by, 139, *150*, 160
Alertness: in anger, 121; control of, 21, 30, 32, 33; RAS system and, 141-144
Alpha rhythms, 139-140, 157; attempt to produce, *156-157*
Amnesia: memories in, 98, 101-104; victim of, 101, *102-103, 104*
Amphetamine(s), 54, 105, 144, 150-151
Amphibians, pineal gland of, 140
Amygdala, *21*; as component of limbic system, 110, 114; functions of, 114-115; location of, *21*, 114; removal of, 115-116, 126; stimulation of, 116-117, *125*
Anger, 8, 13, 110, 113, 121; release of, *130-131*
Angular gyrus, *21, 42*; function of, 42
Animal studies: of body rhythms, 140, 141; of dreaming, 150, 151; of environment, 23-24; of malnutrition, 23; of pattern detectors, 63
Anxiety(ies), 149, 159
Aplysia, studies of, 105-106, 141
Appestat, 118
Aristotle, 9
Artistic talents, location of, 19, 79
Asthma, 129
Athetosis, 68
Athletic ability, location of, 79
Auditory cortex, *21, 40*; function of, 41
Autonomy of brain hemispheres, 79-91
Aversion, 111, 112, 114
Awareness, systems of, 12. *See also* Consciousness, levels of
Axon(s), 45-46, 47, 48, *49, 50, 51, 52*, 54, 55

B

Balinese, dances of, 160, *162-163*
Barasana Indians, of upper Amazon, 160
Barbiturate(s), 150-151
Basal ganglia, *21*; in cerebral palsy, 68; in Parkinsonism, 58; role of, in muscular activity, 58
Behavioral area(s), 10-18
Beta waves, 140, 144

Bile pigment, 66
Biofeedback training: in control of automatic systems, 154, 155-158; machines for, 158; potential applications of, 158-159
Bird(s), cortex of, 13
Birth-control pills, 12
Blackout, *150*
Blind spot(s), 64, 65
Blood lactate, 159
Blood pressure, mental control of, 139, 154, 155, 168
Bobcat(s), 115
Bodily functions, regulator of, 34
Body awareness, center of, 18
Body weight, and brain size, 19
Borges, Jorge Luis, 94
Braille, *39*
Brain stem, *21*; at birth, 23; development of, 19; functions of, 21, 23; location of, 10, *21*; parts of, 10-13
Brain wave(s), *44*; alpha, 139-140, 157; attempt to produce, *156-157*; beta, 140, 144; of different levels of consciousness, 145, 148, 160; measurement of, by EEG, 139-140; theta, 158
Breathing: control center of, 10-12, 23, 30; voluntary control of, 12
Broca, Paul, 10, 11, 42
Broca's area, *21, 42*; function of, 42
Burckhardt, Gottlieb, 125
Bushmen, Kalahari, 168

C

Caffey, John, 23
Cajal, Santiago Ramón y, 53
California Institute of Technology, 81
Camouflage, *62*
Cardiac arrhythmia, 155-158
Castration, 124-125
Cat(s): amygdala of, 115-116; aversion study of, 112; development of visual system of, 23-24; emotions of, 109, 111; levels of consciousness of, 33; pattern detectors of, 63; punishment sites of, 114; rage center of, 109, 115-116; raphe cells of, 145; sleep studies of, 145, 150; split-brain studies of, 81-82, 84
Cell(s). *See* Nerve cells
Cell body(ies), *49, 51*
Cerebellum, *21, 37*; circuits of, 59; damage to, 59; in dystonia, 59; functions of, 13, 21, 25, 36, 57, 58, 59; growth of, 25; learning by, 59-60; location of, 12-13, *21, 37*; muscle control by, 21, 25, *36-37*, 59; programed action of, *57*
Cerebral hemisphere(s): conflict between, *85, 87*; as control centers for opposite sides of body, 80; damage to, 18-19, 80; development of, 19-20; differences between, 18-19; left, 18-19; location of, 13; as

mediator of drives and emotions, 111; right, 19; separate functions of, 18-19; specialization of, 19, 79-91. *See also* Left brain half; Right brain half; Split-brain studies
Cerebral palsy, 66-77; causes of, 23, 66; disabilities caused by, 66, *68-69, 71*; symptoms of, 23, 68; therapeutic aids for, *72-73*; victim of, *66-77*
Cerebrum, *21*; of crocodile, 16; of gibbon, 17. *See also* Cerebral hemisphere(s); Cortex
Chant(s), to alter state of consciousness, 160; of Balinese, 162; of dervishes, 167
Chicken(s): development of visual system of, 23-24; protein-memory studies of, 99
Chimpanzee(s): communication with, 90; effect of lobotomy on, 125; emotions of, 124
Chow, K. L., 98
Circadian rhythms, 140-141
Circuit(s): of brain, 45; from brain, in reflexes, 56-57; of cerebellum, 59; of drives, 114; hot-stove reflex as, 56; knee jerk as, 55-56; of memory, 99, 105; motor, 55; of motor cortex, 58; of motor reflexes, 55-56, 57; stretch-reflex, 55-56
Circulatory ailment(s), 158
Cold, responses to, 110
Coleridge, Samuel Taylor, 149
Collier, Peter, paintings by, *153*
Cones, 61, 63
Consciousness, levels of, 12, 29, 139-159, *160-169*; abnormal, 139; alcohol and, 29, 139, 150, 160; alertness as, 139, 140, 144; alpha waves of, 139-140, 144, 154, 158-159; alteration of, 139, 143, 150, 154-159, *160-169*; amphetamines and, 144, 150-151; artificial stimulation of, 144; barbiturates and, 150-151; beta waves of, 140, 144, 159; biofeedback as control of, 154-159; brain waves in, 139-140, 144, 145, 148, 154, 158-159, 160; chants and, 160, 162, 167, 168; circadian rhythms of, 140-141; concentration as, 139; and creativity, 149, 152-153; dances and, *160-161, 162-163,* 166, 167; daydreaming as, 139, 160; downers and, 150-151; dreaming as, 12, 139, 140, 145, 146-147, 149-151, 160; drugs and, 12, 29, 139, 143, 144, 150, *152-153,* 160, *164-165;* ebene and, *164-165;* euphoria as, 143, 150; hallucinatory, 139, 144, 145, 149, 152, 160; heroin and, 139; high, 143; hypnosis and, 160, 162; intoxication as, *150,* 160; learning drugs and, 144; locus ceruleus in, 148, 151; LSD and, 29, 139, *152-153,* 160; marijuana and, 139, 160; meditation and, 12, 29, 139, 158-159, 160, *168-169;* normal, 139-140; pineal gland as regulator of, 140-141; raphe system in, 145; RAS in, 141-145, 151; regulation of, in pineal gland, 140-141; regulation of, by RAS, 32, 33; relaxed, 139,

X Printed in U.S.A.